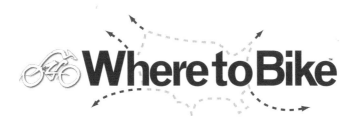

Philadelphia

- City Rides
- Art Museum Departures
- Bucks & Montgomery Counties
- All Those Western 'Burbs
- South Jersey
- Kids' Rides

By Julie Lorch

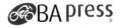

Where to Bike LLC

Email: mail@wheretobikeguides.com
Tel: +61 2 4274 4884 - Fax: +61 2 4274 0988
www.wheretobikeguides.com

First published in the USA in 2011 by Where to Bike LLC.

Design and Layout - Justine Powell
Advertising - Phil Latz
Photography - All photos taken by Julie Lorch unless otherwise specified
Mapping - Mapping Specialists Ltd
Printed in China by RR Donnelley

Cover: Photo by Julie Lorch

Library of Congress Control Number: 2011923125
Author: Lorch, Julie
Title: Where to Bike Philadelphia
ISBN: 978-0-9808587-4-7 (pbk.)
          978-0-9808587-5-4 (box set)

The Cycling Kangaroo logo is a trademark of Lake Wangary Publishing Company Pty Ltd.

Where to Bike is a proud sponsor of World Bicycle Relief.

Where to Bike is a proud member of the Bikes Belong Coalition, organisers of the People for Bikes campaign.

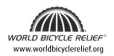

Also in this series:
Where to Ride Melbourne
Where to Ride Adelaide
Where to Ride Perth
Where to Ride Sydney
Where to Ride Canberra
Where to Ride South East Queensland
Where to Ride Tasmania
Where to Ride Eastern Victoria
Where to Ride Western & Northern Victoria
Where to Ride Sydney MTB
Where to Ride London
Where to Bike Chicago
Where to Bike Washington, D.C.

Coming Soon:
Where to Bike Los Angeles
Where to Bike San Francisco
Where to Bike New York City
Where to Ride Auckland
Where to Bike Portland
Where to Bike Orange County
Where to Bike Los Angeles MTB

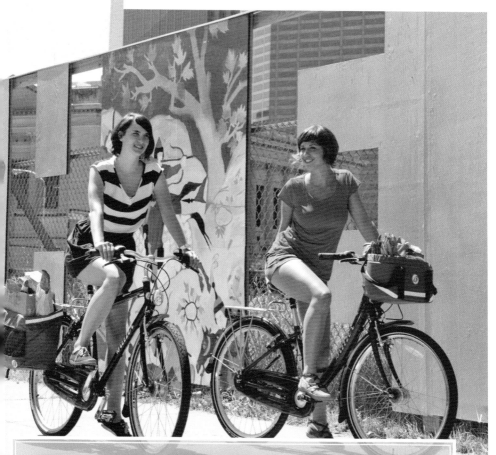

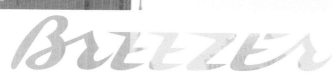

CELEBRATES PHILADELPHIA
The Leading US City in Bicycle Commuting

Awarded "2010 Bike Coalition of the Year" at the National Bike Summit and winner of the Tiger Grant for $23 million in bicycle related infrastructure, Philly is a great place to ride and it is only getting better. As a proud sponsor of the Bicycle Coalition of Greater Philadelphia, Breezer looks forward to sharing in Philly's continued achievement.

BREEZERBIKES.COM

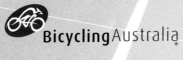

Bicycling Australia

About us...

Cycling has many health and environmental benefits, but apart from these it's a fun leisure time activity for all ages. Most of our small team are active cyclists; we love to ride and hope that we can, through interesting, exciting and timely information, make your cycling experience more enjoyable.

Founded 20 years ago by Phil and Catie Latz, Lake Wangary Publishing Company began with a single black and white road cycling magazine. We now publish four cycling magazines as well as the growing series of Where to Ride guides in Australia, New Zealand, the UK and now Where to Bike in the United States.

We're committed to our vision of enhancing all aspects of cycling by providing information for all our customers. Whether through our magazines or books, we hope to make your riding experience as enjoyable as possible.

Look out for BA Press books and the 'cycling kangaroo' logos in newsstands and bookstores; it's your key to great cycling publications.

We have made every effort to ensure the accuracy of the content of this book, but please feel free to contact us at mail@wheretobikeguides.com to report any changes to routes or inconsistencies you may find.

For more information about *Where to Bike Philadelphia* and other books in this series, go to www.wheretobikeguides.com.

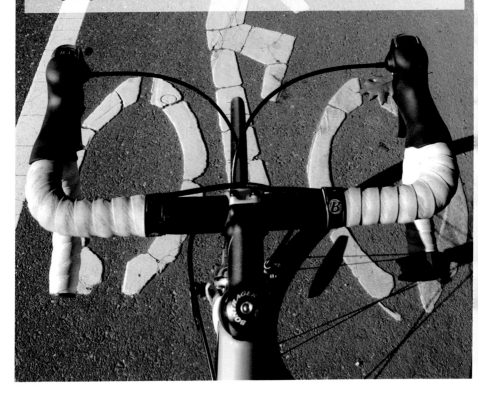

Foreword

WELCOME to Bicycling in and around Philadelphia, the City that Loves You Back!

Philadelphia, home of the Liberty Bell and Independence Hall, where both the Declaration of Independence and the US Constitution were drafted and ratified, is a vibrant city. It's filled with historic landmarks, cultural attractions, arts and entertainment, and lovely scenery in all four seasons, courtesy of Mother Nature. Many of these impressive and memorable sites are accessible by bike. In fact, bicycling is a fast, convenient, and inexpensive way of getting around Philadelphia and its suburbs, whether it's for commuting, exercising, or sightseeing.

Philadelphia is one of a few large cities in the United States in which a considerable portion of citizens are able to live, work, and play without needing to own a car. Thanks to an expanding population of cyclists, a growing number of bike-friendly programs by the Bicycle Coalition of Greater Philadelphia and other advocacy groups, an annual Pro Cycling Tour championship race, and the presence of several bicycling clubs and teams in the region, public awareness of cycling has increased. Safe cycling routes in and around the city are more plentiful than ever. Currently, Philadelphia has approximately 220 miles of designated bike lanes along city streets, with plans to add more lanes and interconnections. The League of American Bicyclists has designated Philadelphia as a Bronze-level *Bicycle-Friendly Community*, and the city ranks in the middle of *Bicycling Magazine*'s list of Top 50 Bike-Friendly Cities. We still have more bicycling initiatives on our "To Do" list, but the Philadelphia region is now a much safer and more bike-friendly place to cycle.

Sincere thanks to author Julie Lorch for generating this collection of enjoyable bike routes. Readers will appreciate the variety of tempting courses to explore. Although downtown Philadelphia lies in a valley formed by the Delaware and Schuylkill rivers and the Wissahickon Creek), neighborhoods in the periphery of the city, as well as in our surrounding suburban counties, provide some hills to climb. Cyclists may choose flat rides, rolling hills, or steep hills. As a Phila-

"Ride safely, and enjoy the sights!"

delphia native and twenty-year member of the Bicycle Club of Philadelphia, yours truly is always eager to discover enlightening new roads for cycling, as well as share "tried-and-true" routes with riders who are experiencing these routes for the first time. Julie's book offers a wide selection of rides for cyclists of all levels of experience, interest, and ability.

Bicycling is a lifetime sport – the vehicle can be adapted for riders of all ages, physical conditions, and if necessary, disabilities. Bicycling is therapeutic – it improves quality of life for the individual, as well as the community, in terms of physical fitness, emotional wellness, social interactions, and environmental responsibility. When riding a bike, the rider is thrust into a sharper awareness of his or her surroundings, whether on a city street or a country lane. It's an invitation to connect with others (pedestrians, runners, equestrians, etc.), and to notice what's around you – houses, farms, city murals, monuments, trees and flowers, creeks, and everything else.

This book gives cyclists a renewed enthusiasm for riding to more places, more often, in the Philadelphia region. Ride safely, and enjoy the sights!

Linda A. McGrane, MS, OTR/L

Gerontologist & Occupational Therapist
Bicycle Club of Philadelphia: Life, Liberty, and the Pursuit of the Ride. President 2009-2011
www.phillybikeclub.org

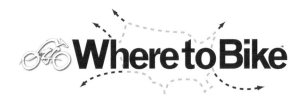

Philadelphia

Contents

About Us 4
Foreword 5
Author's Note 10
About the Author 11
Introduction 12
Ride Overview 14
How to Use This Book 16
Before You Go/What to Take 17
World Bicycle Relief 18
On the Road 20
You, Your Bike & Public Transport in Philly 22
Septa Transport Map 24
Get Involved! 26
Annual Bicycle Events in Philly 29
Notes 272

City Rides

Introduction 34
Ride 1 - Center City Bike Lane Heaven 36
Ride 2 - Spring Garden to the Italian Market 40
Ride 3 - Schuylkill Banks Park 44
Ride 4 - University City 48
Ride 5 - Yards to Dock Street 52
Ride 6 - Kristin's Mega Loop 56
Ride 7 - Northern Liberties 60
Ride 8 - Julie's Sunday Morning Ride 64
Ride 9 - Cheesesteak Ride #1: John's Roast Pork 68
Ride 10 - Center City to Johnny Brenda's 72
Ride 11 - Manayunk Towpath 76
Ride 12 - Forbidden Drive 80
Ride 13 - Linda's Chestnut Hill Loop 84
Ride 14 - Pennypack Park 88
Ride 15 - John Heinz National Wildlife Refuge 92
Ride 16 - The Cobbs Creek Bikeway 96

Art Museum Departures

Introduction 102
Ride 17 - The Loop.. 104
Ride 18 - The Art Museum to Manayunk.. 108
Ride 19 - Schuylkill River Trail to Valley Forge............................. 112
Ride 20 - Boathouse Row to Bruno's.. 116
Ride 21 - Joel's Ride Around the Mainline 120
Ride 22 - Cheesesteak Ride #2: Dalessandros 124
Ride 23 - Fairmount Mansions 128
Ride 24 - Spring Garden Bridge to Bartram's Garden 132
Ride 25 - Dyson's Neighborhood Bikeworks Ride to the Zoo......... 136

Bucks & Montgomery Counties

Introduction 142
Ride 26 - Valley Forge National Historical Park 144
Ride 27 - Valley Forge to Perkiomenville.. 148
Ride 28 - Audubon Loop 152
Ride 29 - Norristown Farm Park... 156
Ride 30 - Tom's Trek from Chestnut Hill to Bryn Athyn................. 160
Ride 31 - The Teeming, Twisting Tyler State Park 164
Ride 32 - Jenkintown Train Station Loop 168
Ride 33 - The Pennsylvania & New Jersey Canal Loop Trails 172
Ride 34 - The Doylestown "Bike for Barak" Ride 176

All Those Western 'Burbs

Introduction 180
Ride 35 - Ridley Creek State Park 182
Ride 36 - Viktor's East Goshen Loop 186
Ride 37 - The West Chester Single Scoop.. 190
Ride 38 - The West Chester Double Scoop 194
Ride 39 - Tom's Ride Around Ockehocking Hills 198
Ride 40 - PASA's Bike Fresh Bike Local Tour.................................. 202
Ride 41 - The Struble Trail & Uchwalan Trail 206

South Jersey

Introduction 210
Ride 42 - Cooper River Park... 212
Ride 43 - Dave's Cherry Hill Loop 216
Ride 44 - Back Roads from Collingswood to Haddonfield 220
Ride 45 - Pie Ride a la Mode.. 224
Ride 46 - The Olde World Bakery.. 228
Ride 47 - Joe's Ride to Nixon's General Store................................. 232
Ride 48 - Long Beach Island Loop... 236
Ride 49 - The Cape May Lighthouse to Delaware Bay 240
Ride 50 - Bilenky's Frenchtown to Easton Tour.............................. 244

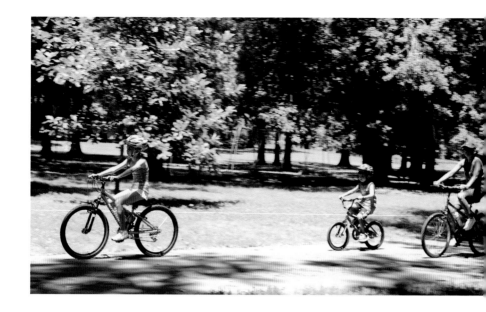

Kids' Rides

Introduction 248

City
Ride K1 - The Fantastic Franklin Square... 250
Ride K2 - The Schuylkill River Park.. 251
Ride K3 - Kelly Drive - Girard to Columbia Bridge 252
Ride K4 - Summer Weekends on MLK Drive.. 253
Ride K5 - Azalea Garden 254
Ride K6 - Clark Park 255
Ride K7 - The Horticulture Center... 256
Ride K8 - Chamounix Drive.. 257
Ride K9 - Upper Pennypack Park... 258
Ride K10 - Gray's Ferry Crescent 259
Ride K11 - FDR Park... 260
Ride K12 - Delaware River Trail (Pier 70).. 261
Ride K13 - Penn Treaty Park 262

Suburbs
Ride K14 - Wissahickon Valley Park... 263
Ride K15 - Tyler State Park - Tyler Drive.. 264
Ride K16 - Peace Valley Park... 265
Ride K17 - Mason's Mill... 266
Ride K18 - Lower Perkiomen Valley Park... 267
Ride K19 - Radnor Trail.. 268
Ride K20 - Struble Trail.. 269
Ride K21 - Beach Haven Bike Lanes.. 270

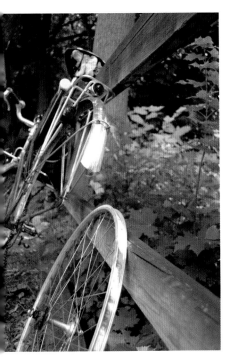

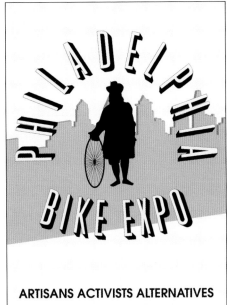

ARTISANS ACTIVISTS ALTERNATIVES

www.phillybikeexpo.com

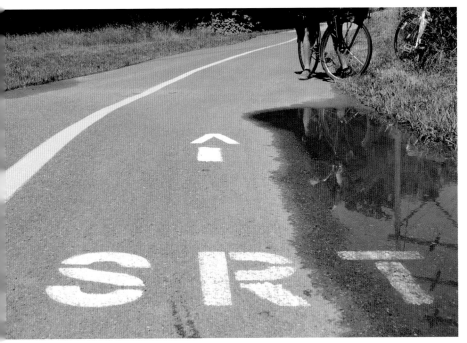

Author's Note

Oh hey! Welcome! I'm glad you opened this book. And please excuse my unashamed overuse of exclamation points and hyperbole both in this note and throughout *Where to Bike Philadelphia.*

You see, I had a complete blast writing this thing. It was a terrific year – turn by turn I biked hundreds of miles, typed thousands of words, and snapped photograph after photograph. I also had the pleasure of meeting a lot of very wonderful people who wanted to share the ride.

While I've lived in Philadelphia all of my life, I grew to know the city more intimately, and more exquisitely, during this trek. I visited beloved places from childhood, discovered new favorites as an adult, and learned to love the bike more than ever before.

But I did grow tired of taking the wrong turn, running out of water, and encountering classic Philadelphia blips such as surprise one way streets, deathly trolley tracks, and weekend parking in bike lanes. I had more moments of realizing I wouldn't make it home until way after dark that I can count. But voila! I took every turn of every ride, and now they are yours. With any luck, you'll be less likely to make the goofy mistakes I did, and more likely to enjoy idiot-proof, carefree riding throughout Philadelphia and its suburbs.

I hope you open this guide enough to make at least handful of these rides your own, and I hope you take enough turns that you'll be able to flip through a brilliant rolodex of images in your mind from the trips you take. Of course there are hundreds of ways to get where ever it is you want to go, and this guide is by no means exhaustive! But maybe it will introduce you to a new part of town, or offer you a new take on an old favorite.

But you know what I really hope? More than anything? I hope that this guide will help you to say yes to your bicycle – no matter the weather, or what it looks like or where you are going. Say yes! It loves you.

Julie Lorch
Author and photographer

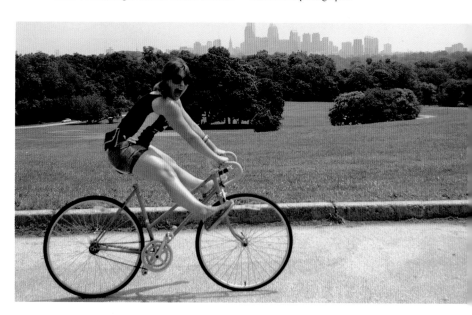

About the Author

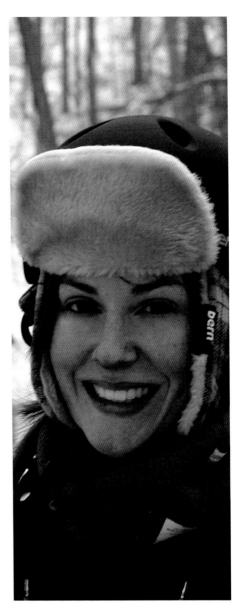

Julie Lorch is a lover of fresh air and hoofing it around the city on two wheels. She often gathers up her friends for an impromptu bike posse and afternoon picnic on Schuylkill Banks. Born and raised in Philadelphia, Julie took up cycling seriously at age 23 and hasn't taken the bus since.

Acknowledgements

Good grief, there are a lot of people to thank! First of all, I would like to thank all of the kind souls who offered me directions during the many times I lost my way while writing this book. I would especially like to thank the good folks of Chester County, where I was almost always confused.

Thank you to all the cycling enthusiasts who suggested cues or invited me to pedal along with them on their favorite routes, including Thomas Madle, Viktor Ohnjec, Jeff Thomas, Dolly Bernard, David Wender, Joe Racite, Louis Cook, Thomas Witt, Andy Dyson, Stephen Bilenky, Curtis Anthony, Sarah Clark Stuart, Alex Doty, Marilyn Anthony, Kristin Sullivan, Todd Baylson, Shelly Salamon, Travis Skidmore, and everyone else who steered me toward their secret nooks and crannies.

Thank you to the Bicycle Coalition of Greater Philadelphia for helping this city to be an ever better place to ride bikes, and for holding my hand through this adventure.

And of course thank you to Linda McGrane, president of the Bicycle Club of Philadelphia, for her awesome encouragement and enthusiasm for *Where to Bike Philadelphia.*

Thanks to the friends who suffered through my constant bike chatter, especially Jesse, Maria, Emily and Jon. And thanks Café Loftus, for keeping me caffeinated.

The most special thanks goes out to my pal Joel Flood from Via Bicycles, who not only helped me choose my first adult bicycle, but also taught me how to fix a flat, always said yes to Indian Buffet, and pedaled along with me for more miles than anyone else on this ride. Thanks, Joel.

Dad, thanks for teaching me how to ride when I was a kiddo. Mom, thanks for reminding me wear my helmet. And bro, thanks for not telling mom that sometimes, at the beach, I ride while talking on the phone and not wearing my helmet.

Introduction

There are cyclists every which way you look in Philadelphia and its suburbs – male and female, young and old, in the parks and alongside traffic. So say yes to your bike and take it for a spin! You'll be in good company.

Where to Bike Philadelphia offers a diverse selection of rides – everything from short, paved paths through the woods to fast city rides alongside traffic, and long, slow rides through quiet farm roads. And there is quite a range of mileage, from two miles all the way up to 51! Whether you are an experienced cyclist or a beginner, totally fearless or absolutely terrified, there is a ride here to help you find your freedom on two wheels.

According to the Bicycle Coalition of Greater Philadelphia, there are over 200 miles of bike lanes in the city and the infrastructure is always improving. If you prefer cycling paths to busy city streets, Philly has you covered – The Fairmount Park System offers city dwellers over 9,200 acres of greenspace. That's 10% of the land in Philadelphia!

But there is way more to this guide than good city biking – there are three chapters full of long, luxurious rides with suburban and rural backdrops in Bucks, Montgomery, Chester, Delaware, Burlington, and Ocean counties, among others. Not to mention a full chapter dedicated to celebrating the Schuylkill River Trail with nine rides that leave from the Art Museum. Plus there's a final car-free chapter just for the kiddos, with a bunch of city and suburban rides good for tiny bikes and little trykes.

It's true that cyclists experience the world differently. A slower place allows us to look more closely, breathe more deeply, and enjoy the details of the landscape more fully. And there is this specific joy that comes with human powered transportation – finding yourself someplace new because of the strength of your two legs is a special pleasure indeed. See what Philly has to offer - pick a ride and find someplace new!

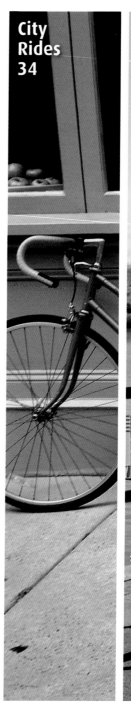

City Rides 34

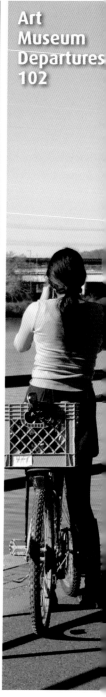

Art Museum Departures 102

Bucks & Montgomery Counties
142

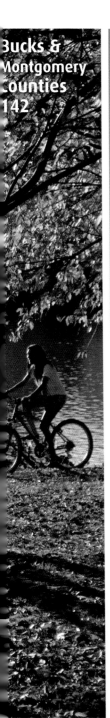

All Those Western 'Burbs
180

South Jersey
210

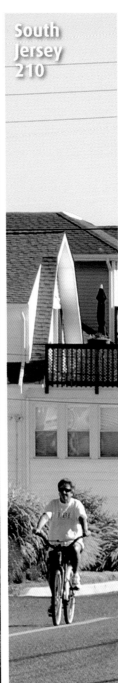

Kids' Rides
248

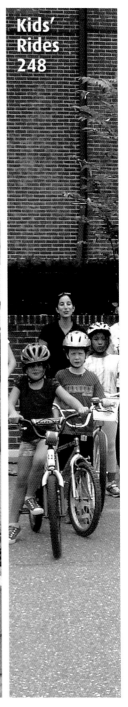

Ride Overview

City Rides

Page	Ride	Ride Name	Terrain	Distance (miles)	WTB Rating	Kid Friendly
36	1	Center City Bike Lane Heaven	On-Road	3.9	2	
40	2	Spring Garden to the Italian Market	On-Road	7.4	4	
44	3	Schuylkill Banks Park	Path	1.0	1	🚲
48	4	University City	Path On-Road	4.0	3	
52	5	Yards to Dock Street	Path On-Road	6.5	3	
56	6	Kristin's Mega Loop	Path On-Road	25.4	5	
60	7	Northern Liberties	On-Road	5.1	3	
64	8	Julie's Sunday Morning Ride	Path On-Road	9.5	4	
68	9	Cheesesteak Ride #1: John's Roast Pork	On-Road	3.0	3	
72	10	Center City to Johnny Brenda's	On-Road	7.3	4	
76	11	Manayunk Towpath	Off-Road	2.2	1	🚲
80	12	Forbidden Drive	Path Off-Road	13.2	2	🚲
84	13	Linda's Chestnut Hill Loop	On-Road	13.6	3	
88	14	Pennypack Park	Path	15.2	2	🚲
92	15	John Heinz National Wildlife Refuge	Off-Road MTB	6.6	2	🚲
96	16	The Cobbs Creek Bikeway	Path	7.0	2	🚲

Art Museum Departures

Page	Ride	Ride Name	Terrain	Distance (miles)	WTB Rating	Kid Friendly
104	17	The Loop	Path	8.2	2	🚲
108	18	The Art Museum to Manayunk	Path On-Road	5.4	3	
112	19	Schuylkill River Trail to Valley Forge	Path On-Road	20.6	4	🚲
116	20	Boathouse Row to Bruno's	Path On-Road	27.3	5	
120	21	Joel's Ride Around the Mainline	Path On-Road	24.4	5	
124	22	Cheesesteak Ride #2: Dalessandro's	Path On-Road	7.2	4	
128	23	Fairmount Mansions	Path On-Road	12.5	3	
132	24	Spring Garden Bridge to Bartram's Garden	Path On-Road	7.8	5	
136	25	Dyson's Neighborhood Bikeworks Ride to the Zoo	Path On-Road	4.6	2	

Bucks & Montgomery Counties

Page	Ride	Ride Name	Terrain	Distance (miles)	WTB Rating	Kid Friendly
144	26	Valley Forge National Historical Park	Path	5.0	1	🚲
148	27	Valley Forge to Perkiomenville	Path On/Off-Road	26.4	4	🚲
152	28	Audubon Loop	Path	4.1	2	🚲
156	29	Norristown Farm Park	Path	5.4	2	🚲
160	30	Tom's Trek from Chestnut Hill to Bryn Athyn	On-Road	27.5	5	
164	31	The Teeming, Twisting Tyler State Park	Path	4.7	2	🚲
168	32	Jenkintown Train Station Loop	On-Road	3.8	2	
172	33	The Pennsylvania & New Jersey Canal Loop Trails	On-Road/ Off-Road	14.0	1	🚲
176	34	The Doylestown "Bike for Barak" Ride	Path On-Road	19.6	4	

All Those Western 'Burbs

Page	Ride	Ride Name	Terrain	Distance (miles)	WTB Rating	Kid Friendly
182	35	Ridley Creek State Park	Path	4.2	2	🚲
186	36	Viktor's East Goshen Loop	On-Road	24.2	4	
190	37	The West Chester Single Scoop	On-Road	14.4	3	
194	38	The West Chester Double Scoop	On-Road	22.9	4	
198	39	Tom's Ride Around Okehocking Hills	On-Road	32.0	5	
202	40	PASA's Bike Fresh Bike Local	Path On-Road	51.5	5	
206	41	The Struble Trail & Uwchlan Trail	Path	8.4	1	🚲

South Jersey

Page	Ride	Ride Name	Terrain	Distance (miles)	WTB Rating	Kid Friendly
212	42	Cooper River Park	Path	3.8	1	🚲
216	43	Dave's Cherry Hill Loop	On-Road	35.8	2	
220	44	Back Roads from Collingswood to Haddonfield	On-Road	3.5	2	
224	45	Pie Ride a la Mode	On-Road	51.4	5	
228	46	The Olde World Bakery	On-Road	42.8	5	
232	47	Joe's Ride to Nixon's General Store	On-Road	22.5	3	
236	48	Long Beach Island Loop	On-Road	38.1	4	
240	49	The Cape May Lighthouse to Delaware Bay	On-Road	25.3	5	
244	50	Bilenky's Frenchtown to Easton Tour	On-Road	40.4	4	

How to Use This Book

In Where to Bike Philadelphia, you will find 50 adult rides through the city and its suburbs as well as 21 car-free rides for kids.

The rides are divided into six sections. The first section includes those within the city of Philadelphia and the second covers rides that leave the city from the Art Museum area. The third, fourth and fifth sections include suburban rides in Bucks and Montgomery counties, Delaware, Chester and Lancaster counties, and Camden, Burlington and Ocean counties. The last section offers rides for kids in both the city and the suburbs.

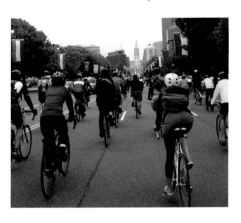

Ride Scale

There is a lot of bicycle territory covered in this guide, with rides heading down paths, bicycle lanes, quiet roads and busy streets. To help you understand the level of difficulty for each ride, the guide has used the Where to Bike rating scale that the publisher, Bicycling Australia, uses for all of its guidebooks. Points are assigned to each ride based on the total distance covered, the total elevation gain, and the road surface and conditions. To find a ride that's right for you, look for the Where to Bike rating in the At a Glance section of each ride. They look like this:

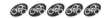

Please keep in mind that this rating system is just a guide. If you're new to cycling or aren't keen to ride alongside cars, then we recommend beginning with the level 1 or 2 rides. As your comfort and fitness increases, you'll be able to advance to more challenging rides.

While the maps have been produced with accurate GPS-collected data, they do not always show sufficient detail to allow you to navigate from them exclusively. The ride logs on the opposite pages provide all of the information necessary to get you from start to finish. Please refer to them as you ride along, and don't forget to make use of the specially designed inside front cover fold out flap to keep you on the correct page.

	1 pt	2 pts	3 pts	4 pts	5 pts
Distance – Road (miles)	<12	12-19	19-25	25-37	>37
Distance – MTB (miles)	<6	6-9	9-16	16-25	>25
Climbing (feet)	<500	500 - 1,000	1,000 - 1,500	1,500 - 2,000	>2,000
Surface	Paved smooth	Paved rough	Unpaved smooth	Unpaved moderate	Unpaved rough

Accumulated Points	Riding Level/Grade	Suggested Suitability
3	1	Beginner
4-5	2	
6-7	3	Moderately fit
8-9	4	
10+	5	Experienced cyclist

Before You Go

Everyone knows that riding bicycles is fun, and certainly cycling can provide many benefits as part of a healthy lifestyle, but if you're new to the sport or hopping back on the saddle after a long hiatus, you may want to check with your doctor about any health concerns you may have.

It's also a good idea to take the time to check out your equipment before going for a spin. Basic things to do include:

- Inspect the tires for damage or anything that might be embedded in the tread.
- Inflate the tires to the suggested air pressure.

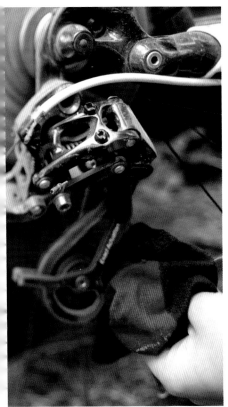

Image courtesy Sterling Lorence.

- Be sure the brake cakes and pads are working and not too worn down.
- Check that the gear cables are tight and that every gear works.
- And last but not least – clean and lubricate the chain. Make sure it's tight!

If you are unfamiliar with these procedures, then pop into your friendly local bike shop for advice or a tune-up. And don't be scared – there was a time when the mechanic didn't know what a gear cable was either!

What to Take

What you'll want to bring depends on how far you'll be pedaling. On most of the rides in this book, you'll never be too far from civilization. But, if you like being prepared for anything, here is a list of items you may want to bring along:

Essentials
- Bicycle helmet with carefully adjusted straps
- Spare inner tube, tire levers, and possibly a patch kit
- Bike pump or gas canister
- Multi tool and any other tool specific to your bike for basic repairs
- Sunscreen
- Plenty of water!
- Snacks
- Cell phone
- Identification
- Bicycle lock
- Cash (a $20 bill in your patch kit is never a bad idea)

Optional Extras
- Light weight rain jacket or other layer
- Camera
- Small first aid kit
- Front and rear lights if you might be riding until dusk

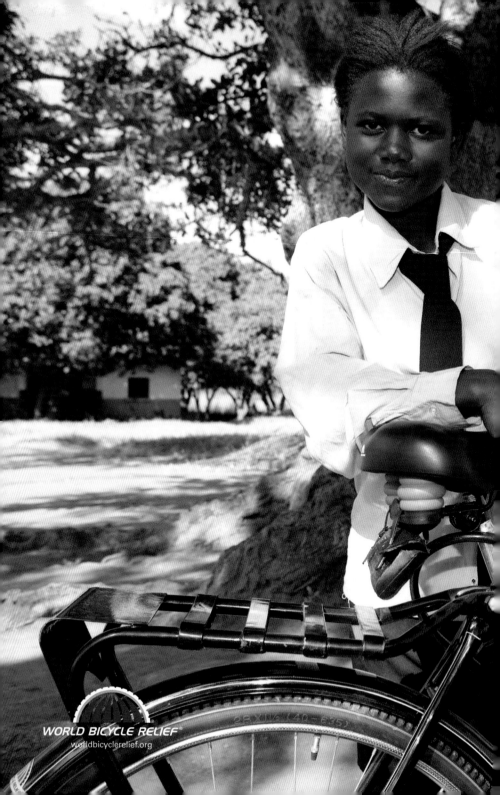

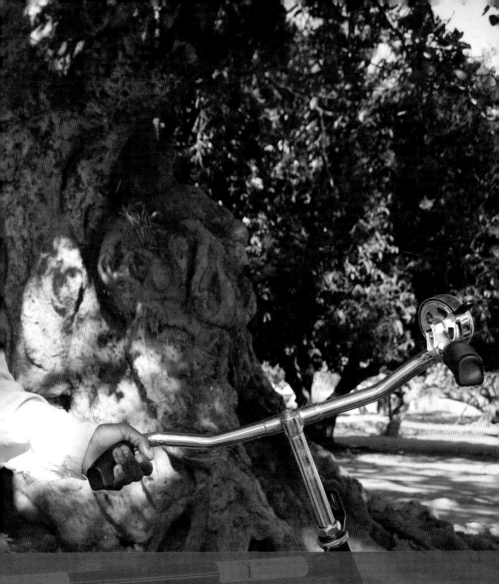

In the hands of a student, this bike is life changing.

Give the Power of Bicycles — empowering an individual, a family, a community and generations to come. In the hands of a student, your gift knows no limits.

LEARN MORE OR DONATE NOW ➡

On the Road

Goodness gracious, be sure you ride as safely as possible! While there are more cyclists riding in and around Philadelphia than ever before (and more infrastructure to keep cyclists out of trouble), accidents still happen.

No matter what type of riding you're planning to do, make sure your bicycle fits you properly. A bell, bike lights, and brightly colored clothing will increase your presence. And always be sure to wear a helmet. Even if you really don't want to.

Here are some more tips to help you stay safe:

On Road

Don't let Philadelphia's traffic put you off riding around the city. With confidence, awareness, and a touch of fitness, you'll be able to claim your space on the road and enjoy being in control of your ride. Pedal your bicycle in a predictable fashion. This means riding with the flow of traffic, stopping at lights and stop signs, staying in your lane, and signaling your intention to turn.

When riding past a line of parked cars, be on the lookout for drivers who may not see you coming. They might open their car door or pull out of the space.

Bike on the right and pass on the left. Watch out for the right hook, when a car turns right just ahead of you. When going straight through an intersection with a turning lane, position yourself in the closest lane going straight.

Trolley tracks are scattered throughout the city and pose a constant irritation to riders. You don't want your wheels to get caught in the tracks! Try to hit them with as close to a perpendicular angle with your wheels as possible. Also be aware of, and try to avoid, road hazards like broken glass, double parked cars, potholes and debris.

On Path

A bit of path etiquette goes a long way towards enjoying your afternoon ride through the park. If the path is crowded, bike single file on the right and pass on the left. Before passing, announce yourself with either a bell or an "on your left" greeting. Cyclists should yield to pedestrians, horses, and skaters. And be sure to ride slowly on gravel and dirt paths; you never know when you'll hit a loose patch.

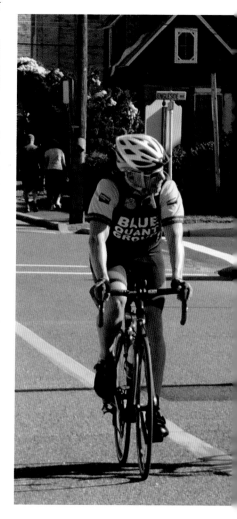

At Rest

Don't let your bike get nicked! Always lock your bike up, even if you're just leaving it for a moment. Grab a heavy U-lock and attach your frame to a bike rack or something immobile like metal sign post. For maximum theft deterrence, thread the U-lock through your frame and back wheel, and then use a chain to secure the front wheel. And unclip all the detachable stuff – water bottles, lights, pumps, even your saddle – if you think it might be at risk.

Remember, you have every right to be on the road. You will actually enhance your safety if you ride with a bit of assertiveness. But do try to be courteous in your journey. In the words of *Where to Bike Chicago*'s author, Greg Borzo, "Wherever and whenever you bike, you're an ambassador for all things bicycle".

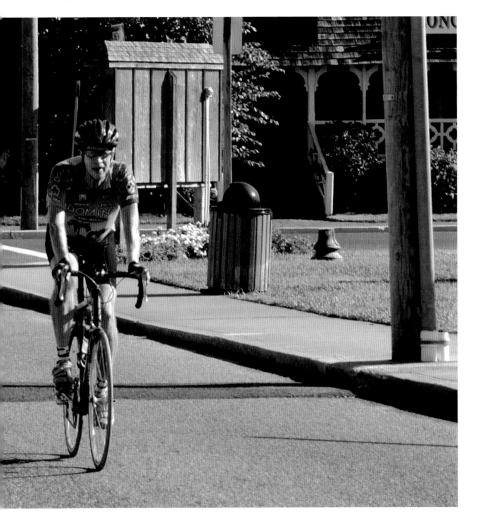

You, Your Bike & Transport in Philly

Good news! There is a comprehensive public transit system here in Philadelphia that, for the most part, accommodates bicycles. Between Septa buses, subways, Regional Rail and Patco lines, you'll find that you'll be able to travel with your bicycle almost anywhere in the region. The system provides you with a fall back to get home in case it rains, your bike dies, or you find yourself too far away from home. For more information, visit www.SEPTA.org.

Here are a few general guidelines, adapted from the Septa Bike and Ride website:

* Avoid blocking doorways, and do not place your bicycle in a space needed for passenger seating.
* Folding bicycles are permitted on all vehicles at all times, but make sure it is fully collapsed before carrying it onto the vehicle.
* Make sure you are able to lift, store, and unload your equipment by yourself.

On Regional Rail

The first time you bring your bike on the train, you're going to feel silly. It's an awkward undertaking. Just go with it.

Bicycles are allowed on Regional Rail on Saturdays, Sundays, and major holidays. On weekdays, bicycles are not allowed on trains during peak hours, which include inbound trains arriving at Temple University, Market East, Suburban, 30th St Station, or University City between 6:00am and 9:30am, and afternoon outbound trains departing from those same stations between 4:00pm and 6:30pm.

There is room for two bicycles in each car in passenger service. When you get on the train, say hello to the conductor. They may be able to tell you which cars have bicycles on them already. Roll your bike down the aisle and head for priority seating – the large, open

spaces designated for individuals with wheelchairs, persons with disabilities, and senior citizens. If the priority seating area in that car is full, you will get bumped to the closest unoccupied designated area or asked to leave the train with a "continuation of trip" voucher from the conductor to get on a train with more space.

A quick tip – try to limit your use of the Airport Line as individuals with baggage often head for priority seating too.

Call Septa (with at least five days notice) if you want to travel in a pack.

On Buses and Trackless Trolleys

There is a rack for two bicycles on the front of all Septa buses and trackless trolleys, which may be used by cyclists at any time. Before you load your bicycle onto the rack, give the operator the heads up. Place your bike in the front rack from the curbside of the vehicle to avoid traffic. To open the rack, squeeze the handle at the top of the rack to release the latch. Lift the bike and place the wheels into the labeled wheel slots, then raise the support arm of the rack over the front tire. The hook will rest at the highest point of the front wheel.

To unload your bicycle, follow the same steps: tell the operator, unload from the curbside or front of the bus, raise the support arm from the front tire, and lift your bicycle out of the rack. Squeeze the handle and

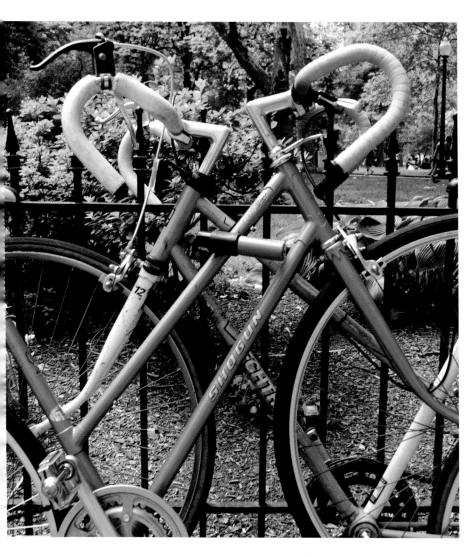

close the rack if there are no other bicycles stored in the rack. Wait for the bus to pull away before hopping on your saddle and riding off into the sunset.

On the Broad Street and Market-Frankford Subways

Bikes are allowed all day on Saturday, Sunday, and on major holidays. On weekdays, bikes are allowed on the subways before 6:00am, between 9:00am and 3:00am, and after 6:00pm.

PATCO Speedline

PATCO trains travel between Center City Philadelphia and points in South Jersey. Bicycles are welcome on PATCO at anytime, but you will do yourself a favor if you plan ahead to travel with your bicycle during off-peak hours. PATCO's website gives the following rules for cyclists on trains: Do not use escalators, yield to other passengers, hold the bike firmly while onboard, and don't ride your bicycle in stations or on platforms. Visit www.ridepatco.org for details.

SEPTA Regional Rail & Rail Transit

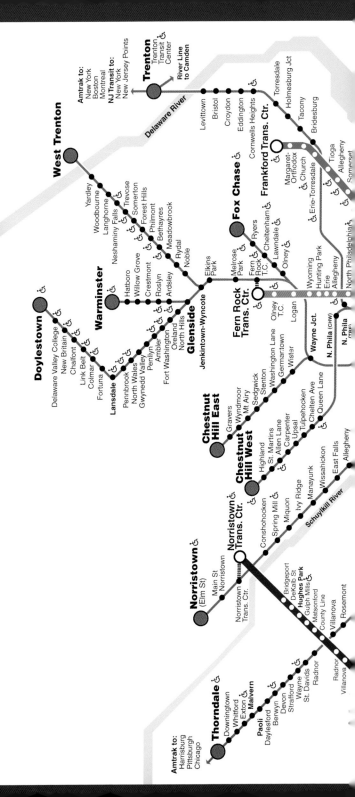

Trenton
Trenton Transit Center

Amtrak to:
New York
Boston
Montreal
NJ Transit to:
New York
New Jersey Points

River Line
to Camden

West Trenton

Delaware River

Levittown
Bristol
Croydon
Eddington
Cornwells Heights

Torresdale
Holmesburg Jct
Tacony
Bridesburg

Frankford Trans. Ctr.

Margaret-Orthodox
Church
Erie-Torresdale

Tioga
Allegheny
Somerset

North Philadelphia

Yardley
Woodbourne
Langhorne
Neshaminy Falls
Trevose
Somerton
Forest Hills
Philmont
Bethayres
Meadowbrook
Rydal
Noble

Fox Chase
Ryers
Cheltenham
Lawndale
Olney

Wyoming
Hunting Park
Erie
Allegheny

Warminster
Hatboro
Willow Grove
Crestmont
Roslyn
Ardsley

Elkins Park
Melrose Park
Fern Rock T.C.

Fern Rock Trans. Ctr.

Olney T.C.
Logan

N. Phila (CHW)
N. Phila (TRE)

Glenside
Jenkintown-Wyncote

Doylestown
Delaware Valley College
New Britain
Chalfont
Link Belt
Colmar
Fortuna

Lansdale
Pennbrook
North Wales
Gwynedd Valley
Penllyn
Ambler
Fort Washington
Oreland
North Hills

Wayne Jct.

Chestnut Hill East
Gravers
Wyndmoor
Mt Airy
Sedgwick
Stenton
Washington Lane
Germantown
Wister

Chestnut Hill West
Highland
St. Martins
Allen Lane
Carpenter
Upsal
Tulpehocken
Chelten Ave
Queen Lane

Norristown Trans. Ctr.
Conshohocken
Spring Mill
Miquon
Ivy Ridge
Manayunk
Wissahickon
East Falls
Allegheny

Norristown
(Elm St)
Main St
Norristown

Norristown Trans. Ctr.
Bridgeport
DeKalb St
Hughes Park
Gulph Mills
Matsonford
County Line
Villanova
Radnor
Rosemont

Schuylkill River

Thorndale
Downingtown
Whitford
Exton
Malvern
Paoli
Daylesford
Berwyn
Devon
Strafford
Wayne
St. Davids
Radnor
Villanova

Amtrak to:
Harrisburg
Pittsburgh
Chicago

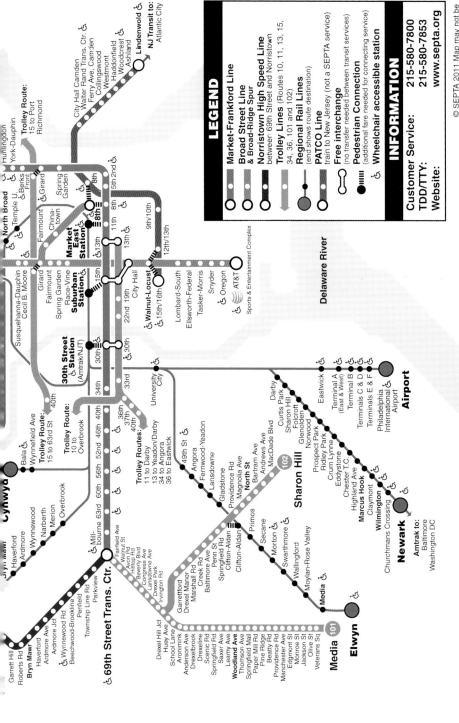

LEGEND

Market-Frankford Line

Broad Street Line & Broad-Ridge Spur

Norristown High Speed Line between 69th Street and Norristown

Trolley Lines (Routes 10, 11, 13, 15, 34, 36, 101 and 102)

Regional Rail Lines (end shows route destination)

PATCO Line train to New Jersey (not a SEPTA service)

Free interchange (no transfer needed between transit services)

Pedestrian Connection (additional fare needed for connecting service)

♿ **Wheelchair accessible station**

INFORMATION

Customer Service:	215-580-7800
TDD/TTY:	215-580-7853
Website:	www.septa.org

Current as of May 2011

A s you read this book, hopefully you are discovering how **cycling in Philadelphia can give you great fun and great exercise**. But cycling can also give people a lot more.

On these pages we'll briefly look at **three outstanding Philadelphia charities** that use cycling not just to give fun and exercise, but self esteem, hope and a practical pathway out of poverty.

Get

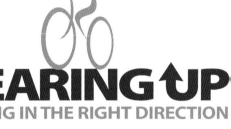

Gearing Up

GEARING UP
MOVING IN THE RIGHT DIRECTION

Gearing Up provides women in transition from drug and alcohol addiction, domestic violence, and/or homelessness with the skills, equipment, and guidance to safely ride a bicycle for exercise, transportation, and personal growth.

Kristin Gavin founded Gearing Up in May 2009. She wanted to use cycling as an effective complement to treatment for anxiety and depression among women.

In its first 17 months, Gearing Up served over 100 women and graduated 25 from their earn-a-bike program.

Gearing Up consists of an open enrollment period and two phases designed to meet the physical, emotional and social needs of women in transition, while teaching the practical skills necessary to integrate biking into their lifestyle. To remain in the program, women must meet expectations, which include remaining drug and alcohol free, consistent attendance, following rules of the road and safety rules of the program, and continued respect of program rules and expectations.

Phase I: During Phase I, women participate in three weekly group bike rides. Group rides begin with a short loop around the block, gradually becoming longer as the women build fitness and comfort on the bicycle. As women track their miles and meet mileage milestones, they receive incentives such as water bottles, shirts, bike shorts, and a gift card. Group rides are led by a Gearing Up program coordinator and committed volunteers from the community.

Phase II: Women who successfully complete Phase I are given the opportunity to continue with the program in Phase II. The primary focus of Phase II is transitioning the women to become independent bicyclists. In Phase II, women enroll in an earn-a-bike program at Neighborhood Bike Works. Neighborhood Bike Works and Gearing Up collaborate to offer a 6-week earn-a-bike course that culminates in the women becoming bike owners.

If you'd like to support Gearing Up, their contact details are:
1213 Vine St, Suite 226, Philadelphia PA 19107
(215) 839-908
www.gearing-up.org
kristin@gearing-up.org

Involved!

Neighborhood Bike Works

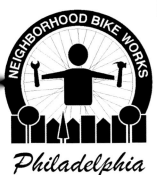

Since 1996, Neighborhood Bike Works has given thousands of kids their first bike, plus the self esteem of earning that bike by learning how to build and repair it themselves. Each child must volunteer a certain number of hours before they receive their bike.

Neighborhood Bike Works' mission is to improve opportunities for youth from underserved neighborhoods in Philadelphia through cycling. They offer free after school classes and summer programs to youth at their permanent locations, as well as traveling to schools, community centers, and churches for out-of-school-time programming. They also offer adult programming at low cost to all community members, and run a full service repair shop at their N. Philly location.

Here's a summary list of Neighborhood Bike Works locations and some activities that take place at each of these:

North Philadelphia

1426 W. Susquehanna, 215-717-3305
Sales, service and repair shop
- Earn a Bike
- Youth Drop-ins
- Adventure Club youth bike rides
- Bike Salon Adult Bike Co-op

40th Street - HQ

3916 Locust Walk, 215-386-0316
(Entrance behind St Mary's Church.)
- Earn a Bike
- Racing Team
- Youth Drop-ins
- Adult Repair Classes
- Bike Church Adult Bike Co-op

South Philadelphia

508 S. 5th Street
southphilly@neighborhooodbikeworks.org
Open Wednesday through Sunday, 3pm-8pm
- Bike Part Art Gallery
- Bikery Adult Bike Co-op
- Bike Café urban cycling information and skills share
- Family friendly group rides on Sundays

Haddington Neighborhood Shop

230 N. Salford, Haddington, 215-873-6696
- Earn a Bike
- Drop in Sessions
- Tutoring
- Bike Church: Adult Repair Co-op
- Group Rides
- Community Service Projects

You could help Neighborhood Bike Works by donating your old bike or volunteering your time, skills and resources.

Of course, all details are subject to change, so for more information, visit **www.neighborhoodbikeworks.org.**

Get Involved!

Cadence Cycling Foundation

Ryan Oelkers fell in love with cycling as an eleven year old when is uncle, champion racing cyclist turned race director, Jack Simes, took him to see the first U.S. Pro road championship race in Philadelphia. Ryan remembers the helping hands he got on the way up to becoming a USA National Cycling Team member.

After retiring from elite cycling, Ryan became a cycling coach, working at Cadence Cycles in Manayunk. With support from Cadence, Fuji bicycles and other key sponsors, Ryan started the Foundation in 2008.

Initially, he thought the Cadence Cycling Foundation would be a cycling talent scouting program for underprivileged kids, but it has evolved into much more than that.

Cadence Cycling Foundation's mission statement is "Helping kids create opportunities through cycling." All kids, ages 9 - 18, are welcome to discover the possibilities that the exciting sport of cycling can offer. These young people learn life skills, such as goal setting, discipline, teamwork and commitment, through cycling. Cadence Cycling Foundation coaches and mentors then provide the resources, guidance, and support to transfer those traits to the college preparation process.

Ryan and his team have been rewarded with outstanding results. Kids who have never even considered that college was a possibility for them, with no family member ever having attended college, have won college scholarships.

Their best known graduate, Leroy Hayes, not only lost over 100 pounds, but rebuilt his strength and self esteem through the opportunity to ride in the Cadence Cycling Foundation program.

Any kids are eligible to join, no matter what their

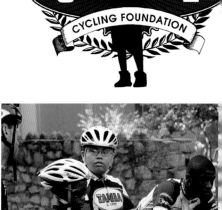

size or athletic ability. They are supplied bikes to train on, and get to stay in the program by attending school consistently, improving their school grades and committing to cycling group training sessions.

There are currently about 14 teams, each sponsored by Philadelphia businesses, with 10-20 kids on each team.

If you'd like to get involved with the Cadence Cycling Foundation, here are the contacts:

4323 Main Street, Philadelphia, PA 19127
www.cadencefoundaton.org
roelkers@cadencefoundation.org
267.973.5821

Annual Bicycle Events in Philly

Bike Philly: A morning of relaxed biking on cerified car-free streets through Philadelphia, hosted by the Bicycle Coalition of Greater Philadelphia. There are options for 10 and 20 mile car-free loops as well s a 35 mile loop on shared roads. Bike Philly usually akes place in the fall.

Philly Bike Expo: A bike expo welcoming riders of ll tastes and styles, this event for "Artisans, Activists, nd Alternatives " includes exhibitors, speakers, and bike fashion show . It's a new addition to the Philly ike calendar, and growing bigger every year.

Philadelphia International Cycling Championship: This is a big, beautiful professional road ace with 10 laps between Center City and Manayunk nd four between Lemon Hill and Logan Circle to total 56 miles. Held in early summer each year, this race is lways a blast to watch – pick your spot early!

Neighborhood Bike Works Ride of Dreams: A multi-day summer ride from Philadelphia to Washngton DC to raise funds for NBW. Consider donating r pedaling along!

Neighborhood Bike Works Bike Part Art how: Exactly as the name would imply: Local artsts make awesome things out of old bike parts for a ilent auction. Oh, and there's a great party too.

Philly Naked Bike Ride: An end of summer ride nat simply speaks for itself.

Kensington Kinetic Sculpture Derby: A design ompetition and a parade of human powered vehicle oats, the KKSD is a fun springtime celebration that ompliments the annual Trenton Avenue Arts Festival.

Scenic Schuylkill Century: Another fall ride, this ne travels through quiet streets in Philadelphia and Montgomery counties. Cyclists choose from 25 or 40

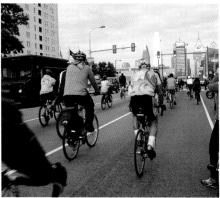

Ride of Silence.

mile routes, a metric century or a full century. Fully supported and hosted by the Bicycle Club of Philadelphia.

PASA Bike Fresh Bike Local: Every fall, the Pennsylvania Associate for Sustainable Agriculture hosts this supported ride through scenic Lancaster County (these are terrific roads – check out Ride 40 for more details!). Hilly options for 25, 50 and 75 miles will get your heart pumping.

The Ride of Silence: An international ride commemorating those who lost their lives while bicycling. The Philadelphia Ride of Silence meets at the Art Museum steps, and takes place the third Wednesday of every May.

Bike Freedom Valley: A fully supported summer ride celebrating the Schuylkill River Trail, with route options between 35 and 60 miles on shared roads. Hosted by the Bicycle Coalition of Greater Philadelphia.

The Philadelphia Tweed Ride: A stylish costume ride through Philadelphia with prizes for Most Dapper Chap, Most Snappy Lass, and Most Marvelous Moustache. The Tweed Ride happens every fall.

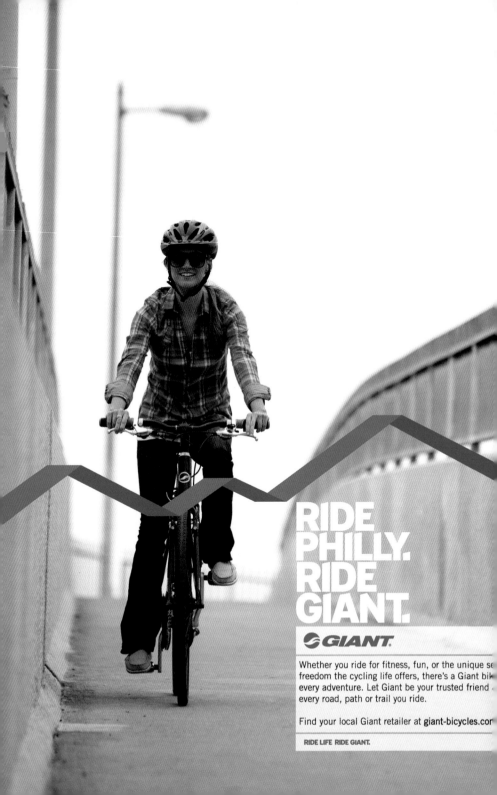

RIDE PHILLY. RIDE GIANT.

⊘GIANT

Whether you ride for fitness, fun, or the unique se
freedom the cycling life offers, there's a Giant bi
every adventure. Let Giant be your trusted friend
every road, path or trail you ride.

Find your local Giant retailer at **giant-bicycles.cor**

RIDE LIFE RIDE GIANT.

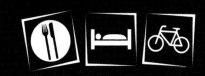
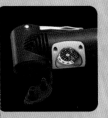 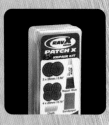 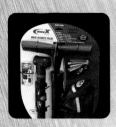 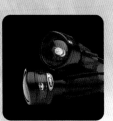
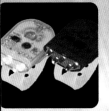 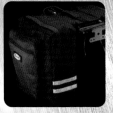 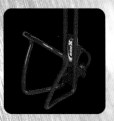 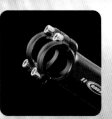
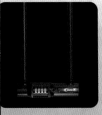 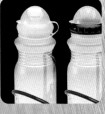 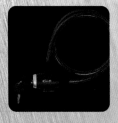 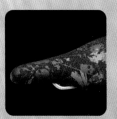
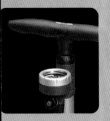 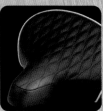 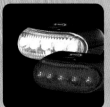 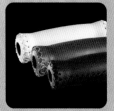

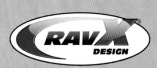

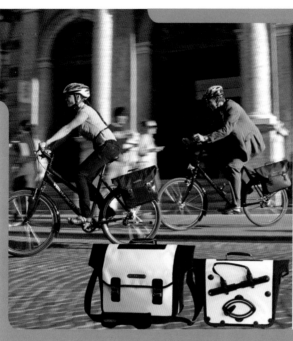
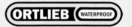
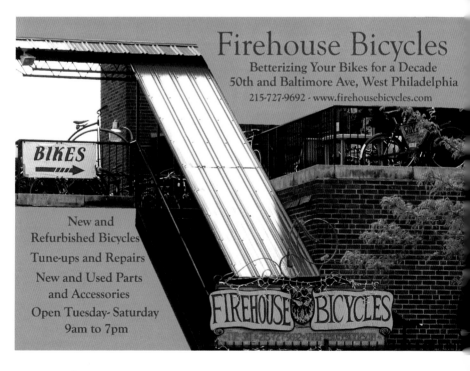

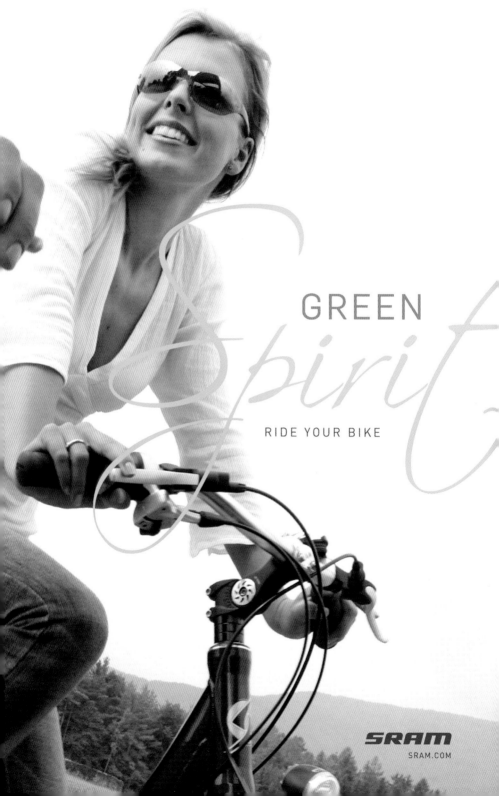

GREEN

Spirit

RIDE YOUR BIKE

SRAM
SRAM.COM

City Rides

The combination of brilliantly diverse neighborhoods and serene Fairmount Park makes Philadelphia a great city to ride your bicycle.

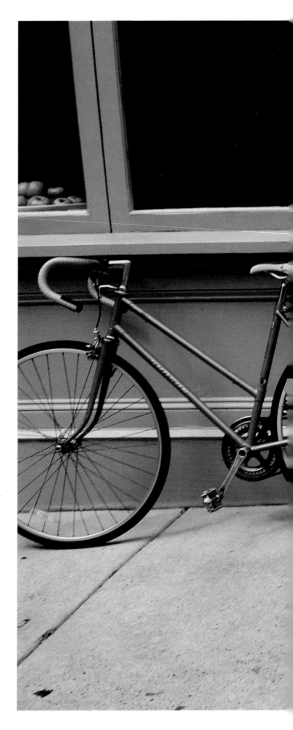

Its public art, history, and dining add to the appeal, as does the 200 miles of bike lanes and the many bike shops to help you on your way. Pedal alongside traffic in busy downtown Philadelphia, cruise through its quiet residential streets, and enjoy some 9,200 acres of greenspace in Fairmount Park.

The rides in this chapter take you all over the city, but it's just an introduction. Many of the rides are short and sweet, designed to introduce you to unique neighborhoods and familiarize yourself with popular bicycle corridors. And they hook up with each other if you wish to extend the ride – in fact, Rides 1-10 crisscross each other so many times that you can take as long or as short of a city tour as you wish. Before you know it, you'll be making your way all over town with ease.

If, at first, you are uncomfortable riding in traffic, be sure to listen to yourself and ride cautiously. Try some of these loops in the early morning hours before the city wakes up (especially Ride 8 – the Sunday Morning Ride). You'll have fun, enjoy the sights and smells that are missed while riding in cabs and trains, and build confidence on the road block by block.

Very soon you'll see why, per capita, Philadelphia has twice as many bicycle commuters as any other big city in the United States.

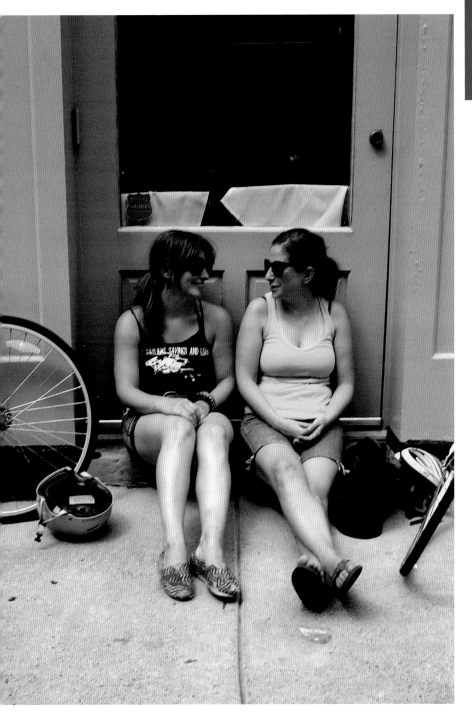

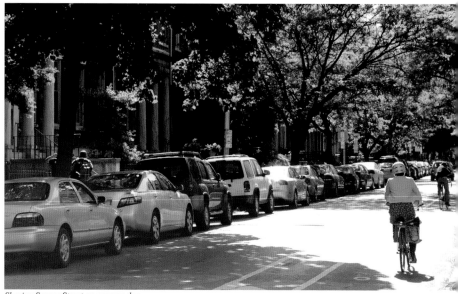

Sharing Spruce Street on a sunny day.

At a Glance

Urban Ride

Distance 3.9 miles   **Total Elevation** 68 feet

Terrain

These new, buffered bike lanes offer a flat, if bumpy, ride through the center of Philadelphia.

Traffic

There will be a steady stream of traffic to the left of the bike lanes. Cars and trucks are permitted to stop in the lanes for loading purposes, so try not to be too upset with them!

How to Get There

From the 'burbs, take Regional Rail to 30th Street station. Cross the Market Street Bridge to Center City and take the ramp down to the Schuylkill River Trail. Head south on the trail and cross the train tracks to exit on Locust Street. Buses 7, 12, and 40 will drop you nearby.

Food and Drink

Nearly every block boasts fine options for food and drink! For a quick pick me up, head to Spruce Street Es-presso – a fair trade coffee bar with large windows and ample outdoor seating – on the corner of 11th and Spruce.

Side Trip

There are dozens of historical sites along this ride, including St. Peter's Episcopal Church, Powel House, and the Independence Living History Center (an open archeology laboratory with artifacts from recent Philadelphia digs on display). The Headhouse Square Farmers Market takes place on Sundays during the summer under the shambles on 2nd and Lombard, or if you're looking for more passive entertainment, the three Ritz Theaters in Old City feature independent and foreign films.

Links to ② ③ ⑤ ⑥ ⑧ ⑨ ⑩ ㉕

Where to Bike Rating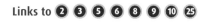

About...

The recent, and fabulous, addition of bicycle lanes on Spruce and Pine allow riders of all kinds to enjoy pedaling through Center City. This is a great first ride if you're just starting out with a bicycle in Philly, or if you live in the suburbs and want to give city riding a go. You'll pass a bevy of cafés and unique shops, galleries and museums, and a seemingly endless supply of buildings on the Historic Register.

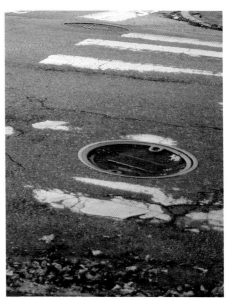

Bumpy blocks around 5ᵗʰ Street.

Thanks to an advocacy effort headed by the Bicycle Coalition of Greater Philadelphia, The City Streets Department and the Office of Transportation installed bicycle lanes on Spruce and Pine streets in 2009 – a major victory for cyclists in the city! The Bicycle Coalition reported a 95% increase in bicycling following the addition of the lanes, which are utilized by hundreds of riders every day.

This simple loop takes you through the heart of Philadelphia. There are stop signs and traffic lights on every corner; please be mindful of all traffic laws and follow them as if you were in a car. Lots of commuters will join you in the bike lanes, but, just so you know, not *everyone* will follow the traffic laws.

We start off at the Schuylkill River Park, which features a playground, community garden, and a dog run. The park offers a lovely green for a picnic either before or after your ride. Riding east on Pine Street, you'll notice that the bike lanes do not begin until 22ⁿᵈ Street. The four or so blocks preceding the lanes are mixed use but fairly quiet.

After you cross Broad Street, you'll ride through Historic Antique Row on Pine between Broad and Nineth Street. This strip was recently resurfaced.

Before the turn around, you'll ride through the distinctive Society Hill section of Philadelphia. Simply choosing between the museums, historic buildings, and walking tours in this area could take the entire afternoon! Please note: if you go exploring some of the more historic blocks, you may encounter a Philadelphia (and Tour de France) favorite: cobblestones.

After the turn on Third Street, you'll pick up the bicycle lane on Spruce to head back to the Schuylkill River Park. The next 20 blocks between you and the end of the ride are urban and gorgeous, indeed some of my favorite in the city. There are a number of excellent cafés on Spruce between 10ᵗʰ and Broad. At Broad Street, The Wilma Theater will be on your right and the Kimmel Center for Performing Arts on your left – both offering a decent selection of weekend matinees. If you're not ready to head home yet, a right on 18ᵗʰ Street will offer a quick jaunt to Rittenhouse Park.

Ride Log

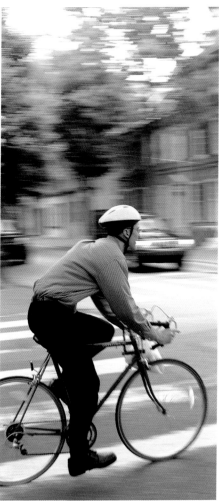

Speeding home from work on Pine.

0.0 Exit Schuylkill River Park on Pine St and head east. You'll be on a quiet, mixed use road for a few blocks before the bike lanes start.

0.2 Pass Fitler Square to the right.

1.0 Cross Broad St (watch for potholes! There are a lot of uneven surfaces for the next few blocks).

1.8 Pass St. Peter's Episcopal Church between Third and Fourth St.

1.9 Left on Third St. Watch for horse drawn carriages.

2.0 Make a left onto Spruce and pick up the bike lanes heading west.

2.8 Ride by lots of places to stop for lunch or coffee.

3.0 Cross Broad St again. The Wilma Theater is to the right, The Kimmel to the left.

3.6 Optional – make a right on 18ᵗʰ St for a visit to Rittenhouse Park.

3.9 Continue down Spruce to finish at the entrance to Schuylkill River Park.

P1 Fitler Square
P2 St. Peter's Episcopal Church, 313 Pine St
P3 Ritz 5, 214 Walnut St
P4 Ritz at the Bourse, 400 Ranstead St
P5 The Wilma Theater, 265 South Broad St
P6 The Kimmel Center, 260 South Broad St

B1 Bicycle Therapy, 2211 South Street
B2 Via Bicycle, 606 South 9th St
B3 Frankinstien Bike Worx, 1529 Spruce Street
B4 Volpe Cycles, 115 South 22nd Street
B5 Breakaway Bikes, 1923 Chestnut St

Center City Bike Lane Heaven

Altitude ft
200
100
0

0   1   2   3   3.9
Distance miles

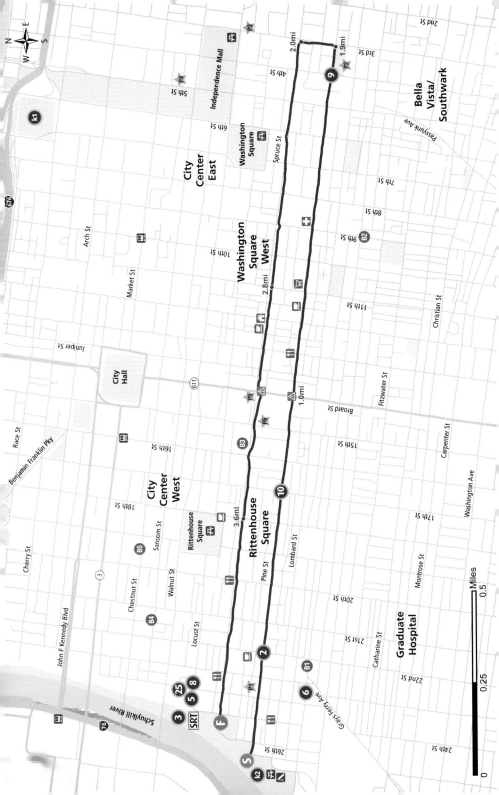

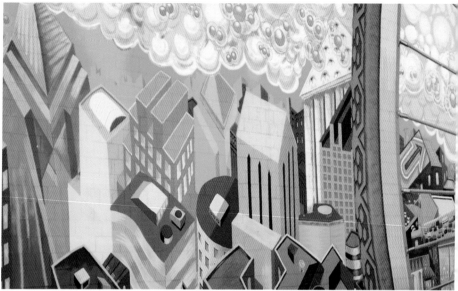

Slice of 'Pedal Thru' mural on Spring Garden.

At a Glance

Distance 7.4 miles   **Total Elevation** 40 feet

Terrain

This ride is flatter than flat! There is a mix of bicycle lanes and on-road riding as you wander about the city.

Traffic

Spring Garden and 22nd Street have a steady stream of traffic, but you will be nestled in bike lanes on these roads (of course, their well worn lines do have a tendency to give encore-worthy disappearing acts from time to time). Columbus Boulevard has high traffic. It isn't perfect, but it is a relatively fast road for north – south bicycle travel.

How to Get There

Buses 7, 43, and 48 will get you close to 22nd and Spring Garden, which is near the Art Museum. There is also ample street parking in the Fairmount neighborhood.

Food and Drink

Oh have your pick! There are loads of eateries on Sec-ond and Third Street north of Spring Garden, the best Pho in the city south of Christian on 11th and Washington, and a number of lovely cafés along 22nd Street. Plus, you'll be riding through the Italian market!

Side Trip

The Mummers Museum, dedicated to the Philly-specific celebration of the New Year, is in stiff competition for the quirkiest spot in the city. The wild and colorful collection of memorabilia and costumes is housed on Second and Washington, just south of Christian.

Links to ① ③ ⑤ ⑥ ⑦ ⑧ ⑨ ⑩ ⑰ ⑱ ⑲ ⑳ ㉑ ㉒ ㉓ ㉔ ㉕

Where to Bike Rating

About...

You'll probably end up in places you never expected along this ride, which, in just four right turns, brings you from Spring Garden to Columbus Boulevard to Christian Street, drops you smack in the middle of the Italian Market, and then lures you up 22ⁿᵈ to meet Spring Garden again. Take this ride on an empty belly – you'll have more variety of restaurants and cafés to choose from than almost any other ride here!

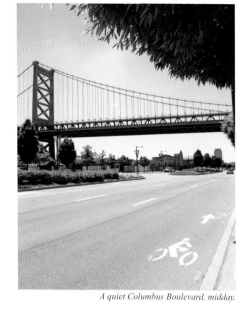

A quiet Columbus Boulevard, midday.

The best thing about this loop is the variety of neighborhoods you'll visit along the way. Allow plenty of time for all the stops you'll want to make – the route edges by Fairmount, Northern Liberties, South Street, Queen Village, Italian Market, Graduate Hospital, and Fitler Square. You'll pass a few museums as well – the Independence Seaport Museum (maritime history), the Mummers Museum (name says it all), and the Mutter Museum (believe it or not anomalies).

Traffic depends on what time of day you pedal, but it will generally be fairly steady. I would not advise this ride during rush hour, as Columbus will be crowded. As always in the city, be on the lookout for potholes, disappearing bike lanes, and scattered glass.

Starting out on the Spring Garden bike lanes, you'll see a couple of works by the Philadelphia Mural Arts Program (there are over 2,800 in the city!). One of particular interest is the Pedal Thru mural on Second and Spring Garden, a 300 foot slice depicting a bicycle rolling through Philadelphia. Northern Liberties is just north of this mural and can be accessed via Third Street.

The turn on Columbus Boulevard may seem intimidating, but the bike lanes will offer some extra space for you to ride (and traffic on Columbus, which runs along the Delaware River, can be surprisingly light midday). You'll pass boats, bridges, piers and the Independence Seaport Museum. There is also a pedestrian entrance to South Street from Columbus if you'd like to meander through Bella Vista.

Shortly after the right on Christian you'll come across the Italian Market, the oldest and largest working outdoor market in the country. The market runs along Ninth Street and, due to its specific blend of cultures, vendors and products, it provides visitors with a uniquely Philadelphian experience. It is most definitely worth a stroll.

As you make the final right turn on 22ⁿᵈ Street, you will pick up another set of bike lanes. Keep a heads up - there are a couple of nasty potholes on this street. Follow 22ⁿᵈ through Graduate Hospital and Fitler Square before crossing JFK and meeting Spring Garden. The slight hill after JFK will keep your legs pumping all the way to the end of the ride.

Ride Log

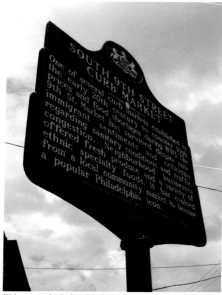

Welcome to the Italian Market.

⭐ P1 Independence Seaport Museum, 211 Columbus Blvd
P2 Mummer's Museum, 1100 South 2nd Street
P3 Italian Market
P4 Fitler Square
P5 Mutter Museum, 19 S 22nd Street

🅑 B1 Fairmount Bicycles, 2015 Fairmount Ave
B2 Via Bicycle, 606 South 9th St
B3 Frankinstien Bike Worx, 1529 Spruce Street
B4 Bicycle Therapy, 2211 South Street
B5 Breakaway Bikes, 1923 Chestnut Street
B6 Trophy Bikes, 3131 Walnut Street
B7 Volpe Cycles, 115 South 22nd Street

0.0 Start out heading east on the Spring Garden bike lanes.

0.7 Cross Broad St.

1.0 The Spaghetti Warehouse has a photo booth! Stop and take some fun shots.

2.0 Make a right on Columbus Blvd (some portions of the bike lanes may long for a paint touch up). Pass Festival Pier – a popular spot for concerts in the summer.

3.1 Pass the Independence Seaport Museum.

3.3 Pass the pedestrian entrance to South St.

3.8 Make a right onto Christian St at the Gloria Dei (Old Swedes') Church. Christian is just south of Catharine and just north of Washington. No bike lanes on Christian.

3.9 Make a left on Second St if headed to the Mummers Museum.

4.2 John's Water Ice is on the right – an excellent summer treat.

4.6 The Italian Market on Ninth and Christian.

5.7 Make a right on 22nd St to pick up the bike lanes. The Sidecar is on this corner - good food and an excellent beer list.

6.0 Cross South St, pass through Fitler Square.

6.5 Cross Walnut St and pass the Mutter Museum to your right.

7.0 Cross Vine St and JFK Blvd. The bike lanes magically disappear for a few feet and reappear after JFK. There is a lot of traffic here. Stoplights and wide sidewalks with very few pedestrians will help you along.

7.4 Up one little hill, and you're back on Spring Garden.

Spring Garden to the Italian Market

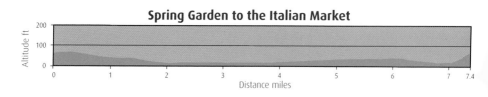

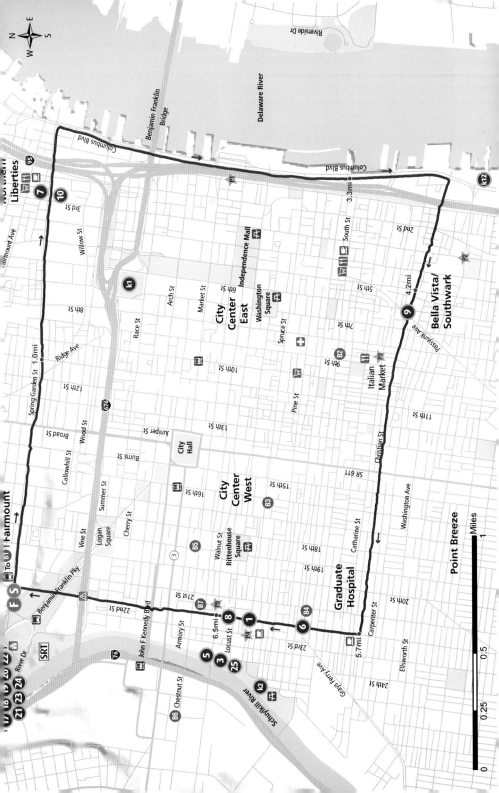

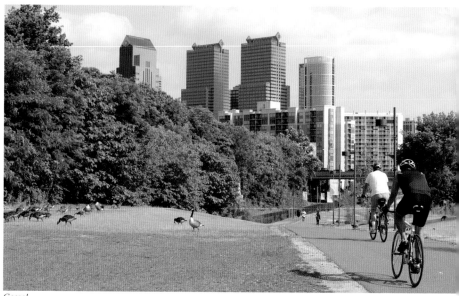

Geese!

At a Glance

Distance 1.0 mile   **Total Elevation** 35 feet

Terrain

The Schuylkill Banks Park offers city dwellers the simple luxury of a paved biking and jogging path along the Schuylkill River.

Traffic

There is heavy bicycle, human, and dog traffic on the banks, and everyone insists upon moving at wildly different speeds! A couple of turns underneath the bridges can be blind, so be sure to ring your bell.

How to Get There

The log begins at the 25th and Locust Entrance to Schuylkill Banks Park. Buses 7, 12, and 40 serve the area. There are access points to the river on Race and Locust, ramps on Market and Chestnut, and stairs on Walnut Street. The trail sits behind the Art Museum, and can also be reached via Kelly Drive or The Loop (Ride 17).

Food and Drink

Bacchus Market is a great locally owned little shop for sandwiches and coffee, located near the entrance to the Schuylkill Banks Park on 23rd and Spruce.

Side Trip

In the summer and early fall, Hidden River Outfitters Kayak Tours leads guided tours of the Schuylkill. Options include the area around the Fairmount Water Works, a trip to Bartram's Garden, and even a moonlit tour here and there.

Links to ❶ ❷ ❺ ❽ ⑰ ⑱ ⑲ ⑳ ㉑ ㉒ ㉓ ㉔ ㉕

Where to Bike Rating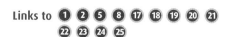

About...

Schuylkill Banks Park is a one mile path that stretches from Locust Street to Martin Luther King Jr. Drive along the river. A well known destination for outdoor recreation, hundreds of Philadelphians head to the banks everyday for fresh air and exercise. You will be joined by runners and cyclists on the path, sunbathers on the banks, and fishermen at water's edge. There are plenty of benches and sitting rocks to stop and enjoy the river or watch the geese.

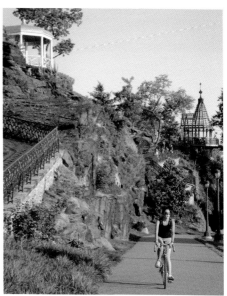

Dusk near the waterworks.

Schuylkill Banks Park is one of the newest editions to 'Complete the Schuylkill River Trail', a campaign by local bicycle and pedestrian advocates to establish a green transportation corridor from Delaware County to Montgomery County. As of February 2010, the Complete the Schuylkill River Trail Campaign secured federal funding for a number of additions to the Schuylkill Banks Park, including a Connector Bridge at Locust Street – a much anticipated antidote for the droves of irascible cyclists who have, at one point or another, waited for the train to pass. Plans for the funding also include a new boardwalk along the river from Locust Street to South Street.

The ride log starts at Locust Street and ends at the Art Museum, but there are other access points along the banks which may be more convenient for you. Regardless of where you enter Schuylkill Banks Park, just follow the river and you'll never be lost!

If you're starting at Locust Street, you'll make a right onto the path after crossing the railroad tracks. You'll pass under the Walnut Street Bridge and then the Chestnut Street Bridge – ring your bell, this turn can be blind.

After two more bridges, you will be in the land of the goose – they seem to love the area near the Art Museum and they do not mind getting in your way. There is a downhill and another great spot to ring your bell around the bend. When you pop up again, you'll be greeted by the waterworks to the left. Boathouse Row is straight ahead, which connects you to The Loop and most other Art Museum Departures.

The Schuylkill River Development Corporation hosts an interactive guide to all the different activities on the banks, including outdoor movie nights in the summer by the Walnut Street Bridge and kayak tours along the river. The guide, which also shows current weather conditions, can be found at www.schuylkill-banks.org.

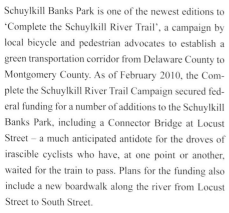

Ride Log

0.0 Start at the trail head near Schuylkill River Park and the Locust St crossing. Ride north towards a series of bridges.

0.05 Pass under the Walnut St bridge.

0.1 Pass under the Chestnut St bridge. Ring your bell!

0.2 Pass under the Market St bridge.

0.6 Geese!

1.0 Reach the Ben Franklin Pkwy entrance to Schuylkill Banks Park.

Now, there are a lot of places to go from here:

Continue straight. Go down the hill and under the bridge to pick up the Schuylkill River Trail and head towards Boathouse Row.

Or, exit the banks at the stoplight. Cross Ben Franklin Pkwy and make a left to pick up MLK Jr. Dr.

Or, if you wish to reach the Art Museum or the Spring Garden bike lanes, you can go up the ramp just across Ben Franklin Pkwy.

Or, turn around and head back to Locust St!

P1 Walnut Street Bridge Stairs
P2 Chestnut Street Ramp
P3 Market Street Ramp
P4 Race Street Entrance

B1 Trophy Bikes, 3131 Walnut Street
B2 Volpe Cycles, 115 South 22nd Street

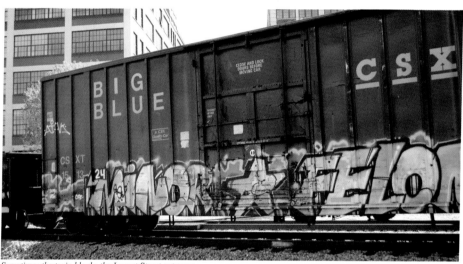

Sometimes the train blocks the Locust Street entrance.

Schuylkill Banks Park

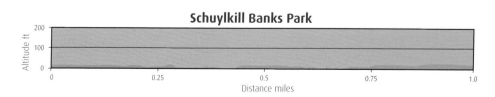

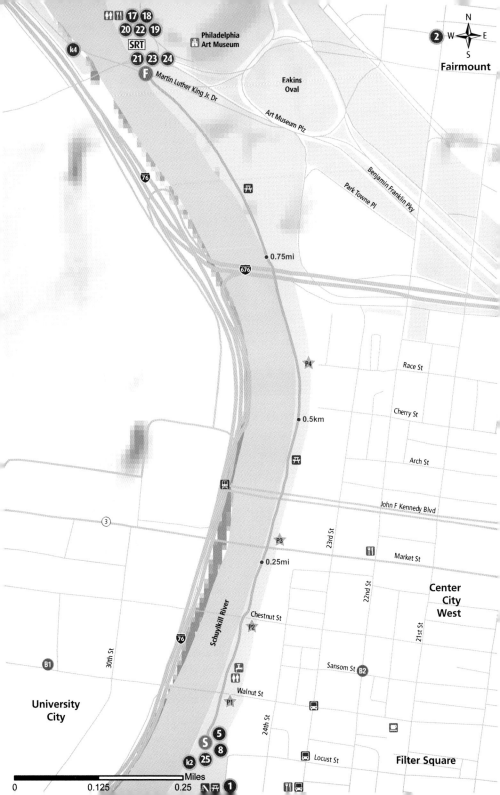

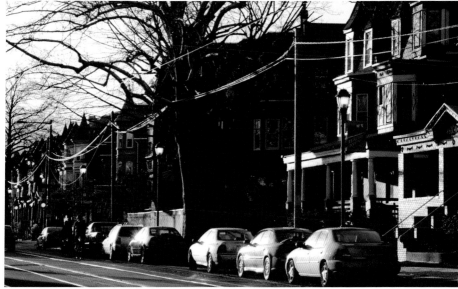

Those trolley tracks are a perfect fit for skinny tires.

At a Glance

Distance 4.0 miles   **Total Elevation** 150 feet

Terrain

This route is all on road, taking advantage of the many bicycle lanes throughout University City and West Philadelphia. Be sure to watch out for the trolley tracks and cross them as close to 90 degrees as you can. There are a couple of baby hills along the way.

Traffic

You will be riding through University City — a distinctive part of town. Some of the streets, including 38th, 34th and Spruce will have a constant flow of traffic. Luckily, these roads also have bicycle lanes. Quiet side streets are sprinkled in lovingly.

How to Get There

Take regional rail to the University City stop and pick up the Spruce Street bike lanes towards Clark Park on the corner of 43rd and Baltimore. Bus routes 42, 30, and 21 will bring you to University City.

Food and Drink

There are lots of options for food and drink along this route – visit one of the many fantastic Penn food trucks, or the restaurants along Sansom Row. You can also park your bike around 40th and Chestnut to choose from even more possibilities!

Side Trip

Stop by the Institute of Contemporary Art on the corner of 36th and Sansom. There are always interesting exhibits, and admission is free. Call ahead to book a tour – quite a deal at just $2.

Links to ⑤ ⑥ ㉔ ㉕

Where to Bike Rating 🚲🚲🚲

About...

Just over the bridge but worlds away, University City has a vibe all its own. Old Victorian homes mix with tiny ethnic restaurants and big shady trees, trolleys whizz by, and everyone always seems to be outdoors – whether it be college kids flooding the streets around Penn and Drexel, friends sipping coffee outside of Greenline Café, or families enjoying Clark Park – University City is one of the greenest, most inviting neighborhoods in Philadelphia.

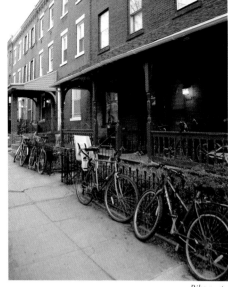

Bike party.

This ride is short on miles but big on flavor. You'll start at Clark Park on 43rd and Baltimore and head north. Clark Park is a fun spot for people watching and a picnic; there are also lots of festivals here throughout the year and a farmer's market in season.

If you haven't experienced them before, you will soon have your first encounter with trolley tracks. They are uncomfortable – riding along side of them might cause worry that your front will get lodged in the track if you veer slightly, and crossing them can be intimidating without practice. When riding over tracks, make sure you hit them deliberately, and try to make as close to a right angle with your tires and the tracks as possible. After a while, this will become second nature.

With trolley tracks under control, you'll ride up 43rd Street and then have the option of turning down Chestnut or Ludlow. Chestnut is very busy with traffic, but is also a fun street with shops and cafés. Comparatively, Ludlow (just a block north) is amazingly quiet. If you take Ludow, please note that there is a median in the middle of the left turn onto the 38th Street bike lanes, not a terrible hassle, but you'll have to navigate accordingly.

After 38th Street, you'll pedal down the Powelton

Avenue bike lanes heading east through Powelton Village and eventually arriving at Drexel Park. There is a little known, and very excellent, view of the Philly skyline from this park. A portion of the East Coast Greenway travels up 32nd Street, which you will take in a roundabout way through the Drexel campus before picking up the 34th Street bike lanes. These lanes will take you through the heart of Penn's campus (if you have a hankering for Middle Eastern food during the week before 4pm, visit the Magic Carpet food truck on the corner of 34th and Walnut – it's a gem).

After 34th Street, you'll make a left onto the Spruce Street bike lanes and head back towards Clark Park. If you have some more time and energy, then head a little bit farther west on the Baltimore Avenue bicycle lanes (see Ride 5: Yards to Dock Street for more details). There are more trolley tracks for you to contend with, but the area around 50th and Baltimore is awesome.

Ride Log

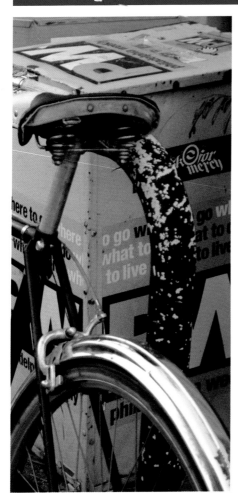

0.0 Start at Clark Park on the corner of 43rd St and Baltimore Ave. Head north on 43rd.

0.1 Cross Pine St.

0.5 Make a right on Ludlow. If you prefer a busier street, you can turn down Chestnut.

1.0 Left on 38th St. Slightly annoying due to the median at Ludlow St.

1.3 Right on Powelton Ave to ride through Powelton Village.

1.8 Arrive at Drexel Park – check out the view and lie in the sun!

2.0 When ready to leave, make a right on 32nd St to head south.

2.2 Right on Arch St.

2.4 Left on 34th St bike lanes. Ride through Penn's campus.

2.9 Right on Spruce St bike lanes.

3.7 Make a left on 42nd St.

3.8 Right on Baltimore Ave to arrive at Clark Park.

4.0 Back at park and end of ride.

P1 Clark Park
P2 Neighborhood Bike Works, 3916 Locust Walk
P3 Sansom Row
P4 Drexel Park
P5 WXPN Public Radio, 3025 Walnut St
P6 Franklin Field

B1 Trophy Bikes, 3131 Walnut Street
B2 EMS, 3401 Chestnut St
B3 Doctor Cycles, 3608 Lancaster Ave

Bike parking on 34th Street.

University City

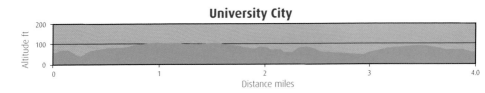

Altitude ft

200
100
0

0   1   2   3   4.0

Distance miles

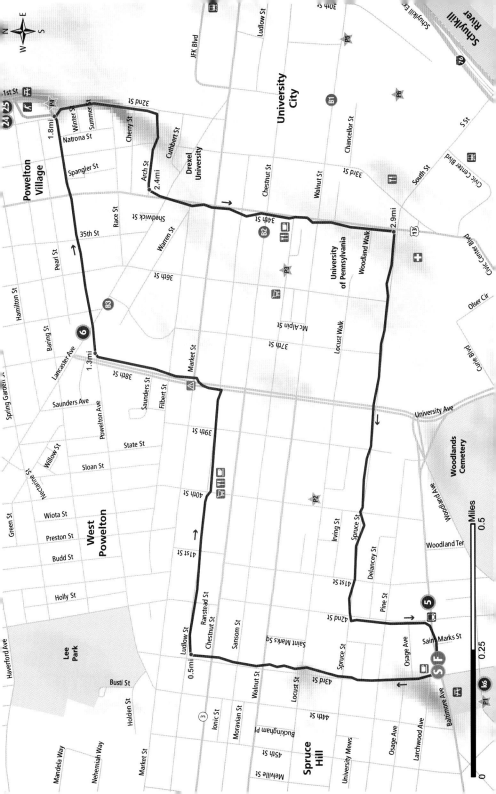

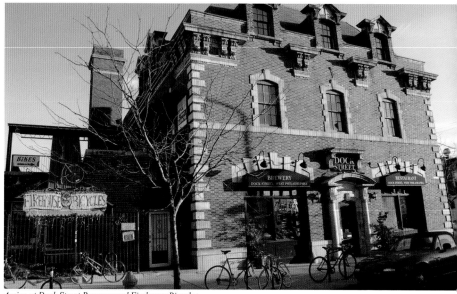

Arrive at Dock Street Brewery and Firehouse Bicycles.

At a Glance

Distance 6.5 miles   **Total Elevation** 153 feet

Terrain

This is a super flat, east –west ride that takes advantage of the Spring Garden and Baltimore Avenue bike lanes, in addition to the Schuylkill Banks Park (Ride 3).

Traffic

You'll be in bicycle lanes for most of the route, but traffic will be heavy in three areas: Spring Garden and Columbus Boulevard, Spring Garden and Broad Street, and along Ben Franklin Parkway in front of the Art Museum.

How to Get There

Yards is located at 901 N. Delaware Avenue, very close to Spring Garden. There's plenty of parking outside the brewery, and Septa buses 43 and 25 will drop you very close by.

Food and Drink

Save up for the "stone ground, hand thrown, beautifully dressed, and hardwood fired" pizza at Dock Street

– it's delicious and a great accompaniment to the beer you'll drink upon arrival. If you're starving mid-way, stop by the amazing Tyson Bee's food truck on 33rd and Spruce.

Side Trip

Two other Philadelphia breweries you might like are Nodding Head Brewery on 15th and Sansom and, up a little farther north, the Philadelphia Brewing Company at 2439 Amber Street. There are tours and tastings at Philly Brewing every Saturday afternoon, if interested.

Links to ❶ ❷ ❸ ❹ ❻ ❼ ❽ ⑩ ⑰
⑱ ⑲ ⑳ ㉑ ㉒ ㉓ ㉔ ㉕

Where to Bike Rating 🚲 🚲 🚲

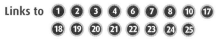

About...

From one brewery to another, Yards to Dock Street is the quintessential Saturday afternoon bike posse ride. This route is the most social of the book by far – the bike lanes on Spring Garden and Baltimore Avenue invite riding side by side and good conversation, as does the portion in Schuylkill Banks Park. After a short 6.5 mile ride, you'll be at the doorstep of Dock Street Brewery in West Philadelphia, ready to share a pizza and a beer with pals.

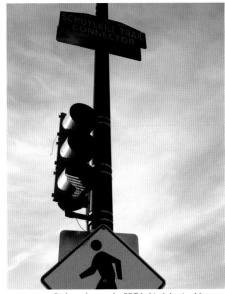

Pick up the sneaky SRT behind the Art Museum.

This one's a winner. You'll start out at the eastern edge of Philadelphia and ride west into the sunset (and a pint of delicious beer).

Hop on your bike outside of Yards Brewing on North Delaware Avenue. You'll want to head south towards Spring Garden Street and make a right. There is high traffic here, so please be patient for the light and wait for an opening to cross.

Once on Spring Garden, you'll enjoy the bike lanes and the company of many other cyclists. Spring Garden is an excellent east-west bike route – it's a bit faster than Pine and Spruce and it stretches all the way across the top edge of Center City.

You'll cross Broad Street and then find yourself in the Art Museum/Fairmount section of Philadelphia. Depending on your enjoyment of riding side by side with cars, you may or may not like what's to come after 23rd Street: you'll be merging with the traffic on Ben Franklin Parkway. There are a lot of bicycle lanes marked here to attempt to get everyone where they should be, but if it's your first time, you might not love it. Stay to the right, as close to the museum as possible, and head under the Spring Garden overpass towards the Schuylkill River Trail connector. You'll pick up the

path at Schuylkill Banks Park along the river and make a left to head south – car free!

You'll pop out of Schuylkill Banks and make your way over the newly reopened South Street Bridge via the Lombard and South Street bicycle lanes. The Spruce Street bicycle lanes (trolley tracks here! See Ride 4 for coping strategies) will take you through the Penn campus before you turn on 40th, where you'll find the lovely Clark Park. There is a farmer's market here in season, as well as a series of awesome flea markets throughout the year.

Just 10 blocks on the Baltimore Avenue bike lanes (more trolley tracks!) and you'll reach your final destination. Baltimore isn't as well paved as other sections of this ride, but it is chock full of interesting little shops and galleries, so be sure to ride slowly and take it all in. An added bonus? If you catch a flat, Firehouse Bicycles is right next to Dock Street Brewing. They'll fix you up while you finish your slice!

Ride 5 - Yards to Dock Street

Ride Log

0.0 Start off at Yards Brewing on Delaware Ave/Columbus Blvd and head south towards Spring Garden (Yards is on the northbound side of the street, so, you'll have to cross Columbus).

0.2 Make a right on Spring Garden to pick up bike lanes

1.4 Cross Broad St. Heavy traffic area – use caution. Continue in the bike lanes.

2.3 Merge with Ben Franklin Pkwy and pick up the bicycle lanes. You'll ride just in front the Art Museum and then make a right to head down towards the SRT.

2.6 Cross Ben Franklin Pkwy at the light and enter Schuylkill Banks Park. Make a left at the entrance to Schuylkill Banks Park, and take the trail to Locust St.

3.6 Exit Schuylkill Banks on Locust. Cross train tracks and take Locust to 24th St. Make a right on 24th.

3.9 Right on Lombard – pick up bicycle lanes and follow the curves around to the South St Bridge.

4.2 Make a right over South St Bridge to cross the river – more awesome bike lanes for you!

4.4 Keep straight on Spruce St bike lanes through Penn Campus.

5.3 Take a left on 40th St.

5.5 Make a right on Baltimore Ave bicycle lanes. You'll pedal for 10 blocks on Baltimore (watch for trolley tracks!).

6.5 Arrive at Dock St Brewing.

When ready to return, you can head back towards Center City via Baltimore, Spruce and the South, or you can pick up one of the many links for a second

P1 Yards Brewery, 901 North Delaware Ave
P2 South Street Bridge
P3 Neighborhood Bike Works, 3916 Locust Walk
P4 Clark Park
P5 Dock St Brewery, 701 South 50th St

B1 Fairmount Bicycles, 2015 Fairmount Ave
B2 Volpe Cycles, 115 South 22nd Street
B3 Bicycle Therapy, 2211 South Street
B4 Trophy Bikes, 3131 Walnut Street
B5 Firehouse Bicycles, 701 South 50th St

destination. My suggested option would be to get creative with your post Dock Street route and extend your posse into the evening.

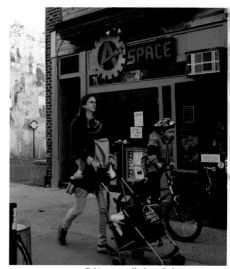
Taking a stroll along Baltimore Avenue.

Yards to Dock Street

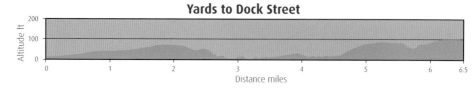

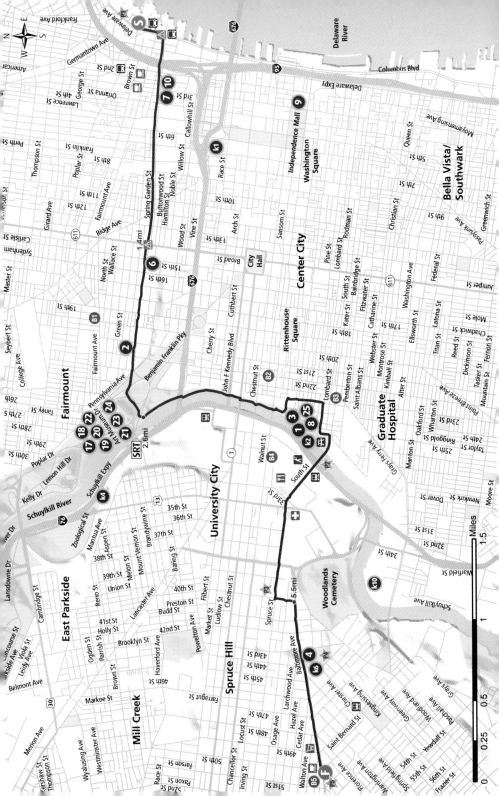

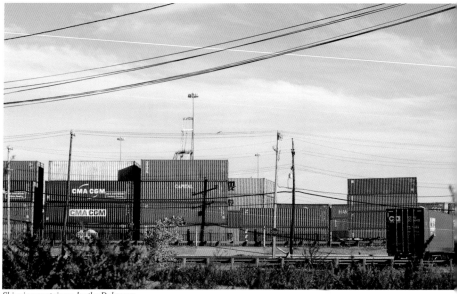

Shipping containers by the Delaware.

At a Glance

Distance 25.4 miles   **Total Elevation** 229 feet

Terrain

You will be treated to decent hills in the first eight miles through Fairmount Park, followed by a flat ride through the city.

Traffic

This route picks up a lot of bike lanes, some streets will have you riding alongside cars. The Fairmount Park section will be on the quiet side, but you'll be pedaling alongside steady traffic for most of the way through the city.

How to Get There

The ride log starts smack in the middle of Center City on 16th and Arch. There are unlimited choices for buses, trains, and subways to bring you here.

Food and Drink

You'll pass many, many spots for a bite on this route.

I stopped at Sitar Indian Buffet on 38th Street between Market and Chestnut. The lunch buffet is basically rocket fuel.

Side Trip

Oh geez… the Please Touch Museum, the Japanese Tea Garden, the Horticulture Center, The Mann, South Street, the Naval Yard, the Stadiums, Love Park… you'll pass them all!

Links to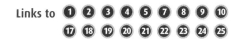

Where to Bike Rating

About...

Thanks to Kristin Sullivan, who biked from Fairbanks, Alaska to Ushuala, Argentina in 2005. Kristin now works for the Mayor's Office of Sustainability, but remains an avid outdoorswoman. This loop is Kristin's take on the city as her playground, and it's neverending! You'll bike from Fairmount Park to FDR Park in one giant loop, hopefully taking in views of the city you've never seen and trekking down paths you didn't know existed.

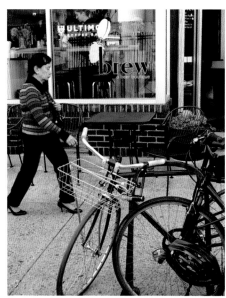

Bikes outside Ultimo on 15th Street.

This ride begins on 16th and Arch, just below the headquarters of the Mayor's Office of Sustainability. You'll hit the bike lanes along Benjamin Franklin Parkway and head towards the Art Museum. For the most part, you'll stay off the SRT, instead picking up a road that will take you over the Girard Bridge and into West Fairmount Park.

Once across the bridge, you'll be treated to a network of bike lanes as you pass the Please Touch Museum, the Horticulture Center, the Whispering Bench, and Belmont Plateau, among other unique sites. This area has some strong hills and a few weird intersections – you might lose your way the first few times you come up here but it's a great place to ride your bike. Make sure to take in the view from Belmont Plateau – it will be an instant favorite.

After Fairmount, you'll head through West Philadelphia via Lancaster Avenue. Watch for the trolley tracks here! You'll pedal inside bike lanes on 38th Street and Spruce Street over the new South Street Bridge, which is beautiful, and then head South on 15th Street. Be sure to take it slow if you're not used to riding on narrow streets with parked cars. Need a coffee break? Stop into Ultimo on 15th and Mifflin. Need a beer? Visit South

Philly Tap Room on the same corner.

Eventually you'll make your way to FDR Park - a big park in South Philly. For more info about this park, see Kids' Ride 11. After riding around the loop here, you'll pop out at Broad and Pattison – a busy intersection. Use caution here.

You'll follow Pattison past the stadiums and through an industrial landscape before reaching Columbus Boulevard. If interested you can pick up the short Delaware River/Pier 70 Trail (Kids' Ride 12). You'll then continue north on Columbus Boulevard, which has steady traffic but whose bike lanes provide a good north-south cycling option, until you reach Spring Garden, which also has bike lanes. Hang a left on Spring Garden and head back towards 16th and Arch to finish your ride.

Ride Log

0.0 Start out on 16th and Ben Franklin Pkwy, head towards the Art Museum in the parkway's bike lanes.

1.5 Make a right onto Poplar, heading away from Lloyd Hall.

1.6 Left on W Sedgley Dr and head towards Girard Bridge.

2.0 Left on Brewery Hill Dr to cross Girard (caution, please!).

2.2 Post bridge, make a right onto Lansdowne Dr.

2.4 Right on Sweet Briar and follow bike path to the left.

3.1 Pick up Black Rd and follow it until you reach Lansdowne Dr (again).

3.5 Make a tight right at Lansdowne, you'll pass the Please Touch Museum.

3.8 Right on Belmont Dr (follow signs for Japanese Tea House), then a quick right on Horticultural Dr to loop around the Horticulture Center.

4.3 Right on Belmont Dr (caution crossing Montgomery Dr). Climb the hill to the plateau!

5.1 After the mansion, make a right on Chamounix Dr.

5.7 Left on Ford Rd.

6.3 Left on Monument Rd.

6.8 Make a right and then bear left on Georges Hill Dr. Big downhill here.

7.0 Left on Georges Hill Dr, and enjoy the downhill.

8.0 Bear right towards S Concourse St.

8.5 Right on Belmont Ave.

9.4 Left on Lancaster Ave, heading towards Center City (watch out for trolley tracks!).

10.2 Right on 38th St.

10.8 Left on Spruce St, follow until it becomes South St.

11.6 Cross the new South St Bridge! Pick up South St

bike lanes, which end abruptly, but it's a nice gesture.

12.6 Right on 15th St – narrow and with street parking.

14.5 Right on Oregon Ave.

14.9 Left on 20th St. Take 20th all the way to FDR Park.

15.7 Follow the FDR path around The Lakes.

17.1 Exit FDR at Pattison and Broad. Cross Broad (caution!) and head East on Pattison.

18.8 After the stadiums, Pattison becomes Columbus Blvd. Look for bike lanes here.

20.5 If you want to check out the new Pier 70 trail along the Delaware, hang a right into the Walmart parking lot. The trail starts behind the store and ends at Washington Ave. If not, stay on Columbus.

23.4 Left on Spring Garden.

24.8 Left on 15th St.

25.3 Right on Arch.

25.4 Back to the start by Love Park.

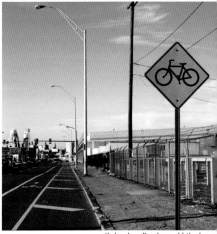

Columbus Boulevard bike lanes

Kristin's Mega Loop

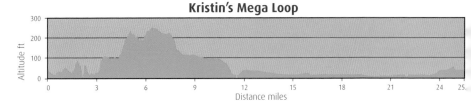

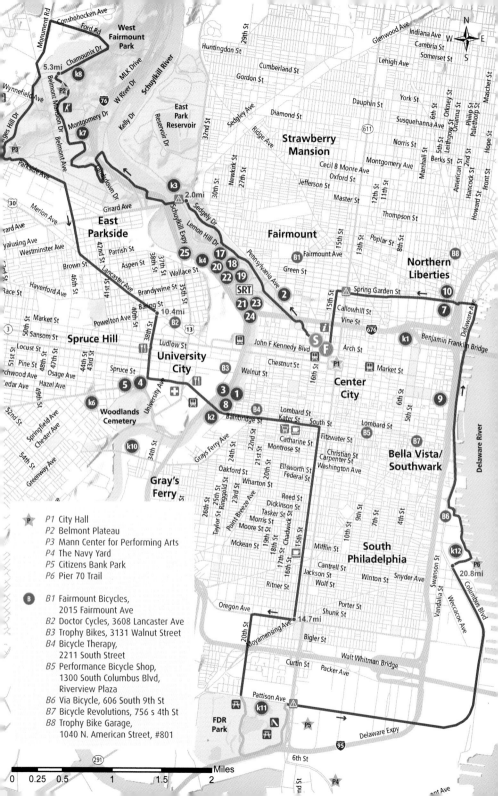

Northern Liberties Ride 7

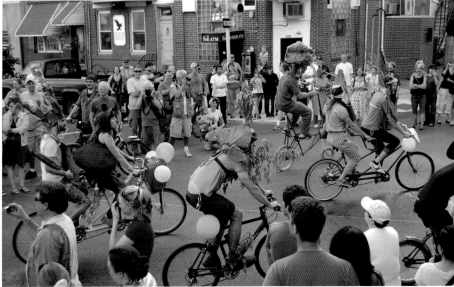

2010 Kensington Kinetic Sculpture Derby.   *Photo courtesy Bike Coaltion of Greater Philadelphia*

At a Glance

Distance 5.1 miles   **Total Elevation** 80 feet

Terrain

You'll weave in and out of bike lanes as you ride on-road all the way to Penn Treaty Park and back. There's one, short hill on Second Street in Northern Liberties.

Traffic

Traffic will be heavy on most streets, including Second and Sixth, Columbus Boulevard, Girard, and Market. There are bicycle lanes on Columbus, Spring Garden, and Sixth Street.

How to Get There

The ride begins at the corner of Fifth and Market. If coming from the 'burbs, take regional rail to Market East station and tote your bike from the 10th and Market exit on down to Fifth. Additionally, busses 17, 33, 48, and 57 all stop at Fourth and Market.

Food and Drink

Lock up the bikes and grab a bite on Second Street in

Northern Liberties. There are so many little cafés and restaurants in this area, including plenty of options for outdoor dining and a mid-ride beer. Standard Tap and Cantina Dos Segundos, both around Second and Poplar, are tried and true favorites.

Side Trip

You might want to check out the Kensington Kinetic Sculpture Derby, which takes place every spring and travels through Penn Treaty Park. It's a parade and celebration of human powered transportation with crazy looking, handmade floats. For more, check out www kinetickensington.com.

Links to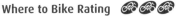

Where to Bike Rating

About...

Bike from Old City to Penn Treaty and take a stroll through Northern Liberties in between! Nolibs is another one of those unique Philadelphia neighborhoods packed with shops, cafés, and galleries. There are also a few open spaces that are terrific for public sitting and people-watching. But you'll have to be comfortable riding in traffic – these roads have a steady stream of cars and bikes!

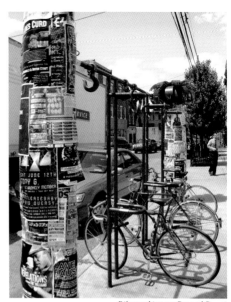

Bike parking on Second Street.

Start out on Fifth and Market and decide how you feel – you can head straight north in the Fifth Street bicycle lane (see rides 8 and 10 for details) or make your way down to Third Street. Fifth will have faster traffic but a bicycle lane, Third offers a classic Philadelphia cityscape, with small businesses and brightly painted signs scattered about its brick buildings, but the street is a bit narrow.

Whether you take Third or Fifth, you'll end up on the Spring Garden bike lanes and make a right towards the Delaware River and a left on the Columbus Avenue bike lanes towards Penn Treaty Park. There will be heavy traffic on this corner, so take your time and stick to those bike lanes as you head north. If you want to skip Penn Treaty Park, then just keep on Third Street and make your way onto Northern Liberties.

Soon you will arrive at Penn Treaty Park! What is this place? It's the site believed to be where William Penn and Lenape Chief Tamanend entered into a Treaty of Friendship under a great elm tree, in 1682. The spot was commemorated by an obelisk in 1827, after the original elm fell. Philadelphia's old!

After you leave Penn Treaty, you'll make your way over to Northern Liberties via East Allen Street, Frankford and Girard. The turn on Second Street might be a hassle – you'll have to get into the left lane and cross some trolley tracks to make it happen, but there's a lot to do on Second – lock up your bikes and have a stroll! Stop by the Piazza, a large public space (with a huge outdoor screen that shows Phillies games, among other programming) and Liberties Walk on your way through Nolibs.

Heading home is simple – make a right at the 700 Club on Fairmount Avenue and then a left on the Sixth Street bicycle lanes. Try not to blow through the red lights here, because some of these intersections are blind and quite busy. Pass Franklin Square (Kids' Ride 1) and before you know it, you're back to the start.

Side note: Don't miss the Liberty Bell, nestled in the corner of Sixth and Market. The National Constitution Center and Independence Hall are also right here, if you are interested in learning more about, you know... the birth of our nation.

Ride Log

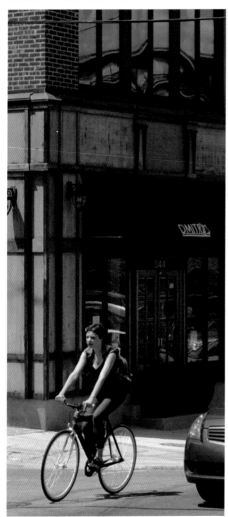

Easy riding around Northern Liberties.

0.0 Start on Fifth and Market. Bike down Market and make a left to head north on Third St. If you prefer a bike lane, try heading north on Fifth St instead.

0.8 Right on Spring Garden.

1.2 Left on Columbus Blvd bike lanes – use caution on this turn. High traffic area!

1.8 Arrive at Penn Treaty Park! Hang out.

1.9 After leaving Penn Treaty, cross Columbus Blvd and make a quick left on E Allen St. It's the first street parallel to Columbus.

2.3 Right on Frankford Ave.

2.5 Left on Girard Ave. Trolley tracks here!

2.8 Left on N Second St and cruise through the center of Northern Liberties, all the way down to Fairmount Ave.

3.2 Make a right on Fairmount Ave.

3.6 Left on N Sixth St bike lanes.

3.9 Pedal through 676 underpass, then wait at the light and follow the traffic pattern. This can be a tricky corner to negotiate!

4.5 Left on Market St.

5.1 Arrive at the beginning.

P1 Independence Hall
P2 Penn Treaty Park
P3 The Piazza at Schmidts
P4 Franklin Square
P5 National Constitution Center
P6 The Liberty Bell

B1 Jay's Pedal Power, 512 East Girard Ave
B2 Bicycle Stable, 1420 Frankford Ave
B3 Trophy Bike Garage,
1040 N. American Street, #801

Northern Liberties

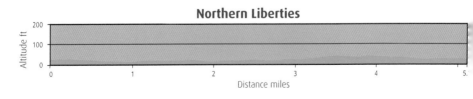

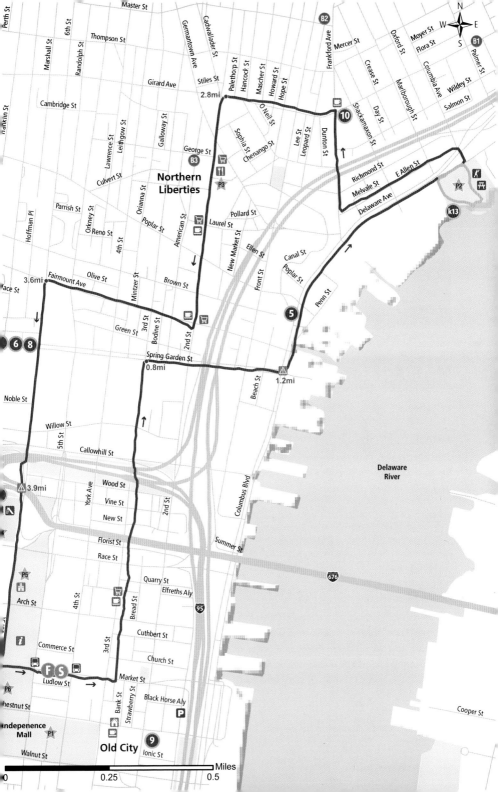

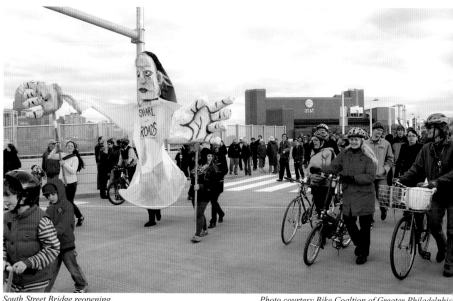

South Street Bridge reopening.

Photo courtesy Bike Coaltion of Greater Philadelphia

At a Glance

Distance 9.5 miles   **Total Elevation** 53 feet

Terrain

This is a city ride, through crowded city streets, with lots to look at absolutely everywhere you turn your head, and even more potholes.

Traffic

Heavy. Unless you are an experienced city rider, this is a loop for an early Sunday morning, long before the city wakes up.

How to Get There

The ride log begins at the entrance to Schuylkill River Park, on 25th and Locust. If coming from the burbs, take Regional Rail to 30th Street station, cross the Market Street Bridge towards Center City and take the ramp towards the Schuylkill River Trail. Septa buses 7,12 and 40 will drop you nearby.

Food and Drink

Almost every street will have options for you. High-

lights include cafés around Rittenhouse square, Pho 7 on Washington Avenue, Sabrina's in the Italian Market on Ninth and Christian, and the portions along South and 18th streets. You'll ride through Chinatown, too!

Side Trip

The opportunities for people-watching and public sitting throughout this loop are pretty great – you'll want to park your bike and hang out on almost every corner of this ride (I do!). Rittenhouse Square, Independence Mall, City Hall, Love Park, Logan Square, and the Art Museum steps are just a few of the stops.

Links to ① ② ③ ⑤ ⑥ ⑦ ⑨ ⑩ ⑰
⑱ ⑲ ⑳ ㉑ ㉒ ㉓ ㉔ ㉕

Where to Bike Rating

About...

These are some of my favorite streets in the city – in my opinion, this route showcases the best stuff to see from a bike in Philadelphia. The buildings flutter between old and new, serene open spaces are jammed into a hustling city, ethnic neighborhoods appear to pop up out of nowhere, and it finishes off with a short stretch along that gorgeous Schuylkill River. If you don't like weaving in and out of traffic, then make this trip early on a Sunday morning.

Nice new lanes on South Street.

There are a million ways to get from place to place in Philadelphia, but for some reason, I always come back to these roads. There may or may not be bicycle lanes, potholes, heavy traffic, annoying drivers, confusing lights and awkward pedestrians, but man, I love the way these streets look and feel from a bicycle.

You'll begin at Schuylkill River Park and bike through beautiful brick homes in Fitler Square. Then make a couple of left turns at Rittenhouse Square to hug the perimeter of the park along Locust. This is an area where bikes almost always have the ability to beat cars. You'll continue to Broad Street and then race southbound to Washington. Broad is going to be busy.

Take Washington through the beginning of the Vietnamese section of Philadelphia and then turn up Ninth Street straight through the Italian Market. This will be super cramped, but also awesome. Continue up Ninth all the way to South through Bella Vista. You'll also pass my go-to bike shop – Via Bikes on Ninth and South.

But wait there's so much more! You'll ride along busy South Street and up Fifth Street through the tunnel to Spring Garden. The whole reason for this is so you can bike south on 10th Street – which is right

through the Chinatown arches. Take it slowly here!

After 10th, hop on Market towards City Hall and make a couple of lefts to ride around the perimeter, much like you did for Rittenhouse Square. City Hall is beautiful, by the way. You'll end up southbound on 15th Street and then hang a right on Walnut through the heart of Center City. If you want to skip this short portion, which swings through 18th Street and Chestnut Street, then stay on Market to 16th Street and make a right to pick up the log at mile 7.2 (at the Arch/Ben Franklin/16th Street intersection).

Benjamin Franklin Parkway bicycle lanes are next! Ride around the fountain at Logan Square and head down the parkway towards the Art Museum. You'll loop halfway around Eakins Oval to bike past the museum and head towards the river trail. Once at Schuylkill Banks, make a left to end your fantastic ride along the river and back to the Locust Street entrance.

Ride Log

0.0 Start 25th and Locust, by the entrance to Schuylkill Banks Park. Head east on Locust.

0.4 Come to the edge of Rittenhouse Park. Make a right at the light and follow Locust around the south end of the park.

0.6 Left on 18th St at the light, then a quick right at the next right to stay on Locust.

1.0 Right on Broad St to head south. If you don't want to ride on Broad or Washington, then stay on Locust through the Gayborhood until you reach Fifth St. Pick up the ride log at mile 3.2.

1.7 Left on Washington Ave bicycle lanes.

2.0 Pass Pho 75. Yum. Soup and Vietnamese coffee, only.

2.2 Left on Ninth St to pedal through the Italian Market.

2.7 Right on South St.

3.0 Left on Fifth St.

3.2 Come to Fifth and Locust. If coming from Locust, make a left onto Fifth St.

3.4 Pass Independence Mall.

3.6 Cross Market St and pick up the Fifth St bicycle lanes. Sail through the tunnel on your way up north!

4.4 Left on Spring Garden bicycle lanes.

4.8 Left on N 10th St.

5.2 Ride southbound through Chinatown!

5.6 Right on Market St.

5.9 Hit City Hall and make a right on Juniper St.

6.0 Left on Filbert to go around the City Hall block.

6.1 Left on 16th St.

6.4 Right on Walnut St to pedal through Philadelphia's (short but sweet) lux shopping district.

6.6 Right on 18th St. Watch for potholes on this one!

6.8 Right on Chestnut St.

7.0 Left on 16th St.

7.2 Come to the Arch/Benjamin Franklin/16th St intersection. Make a right on Ben Franklin Pkwy at the light and pick up the bicycle lanes.

7.5 Follow the bike lanes around Logan Circle and keep heading down the parkway towards the museum.

8.2 Bear left to snake in front of the museum. Make your way over to the right lane and, after you pass the museum, pedal under the overpass towards the river. See the sign pointing you to the Schuylkill Banks Park. Cross Ben Franklin Pkwy at the light and make a left onto the bike path.

8.9 Pass Race St entrance to the bike path.

9.4 Pedal under the Walnut St Bridge.

9.5 Arrive at the end of Schuylkill Banks Park and the entrance at 25th and Locust.

P1 Rittenhouse Square
P2 Washington Square Park
P3 Fifth St Bicycle Tunnel
P4 City Hall
P5 Love Park

B1 Bicycle Therapy, 2211 South Street
B2 Frankinstien Bike Worx, 1529 Spruce Street
B3 Via Bicycle, 606 South 9th St
B4 Breakaway Bikes, 1923 Chestnut Street
B5 Volpe Cycles, 115 South 22nd Street
B6 Fairmount Bicycles, 2015 Fairmount Ave

Julie's Sunday Morning Ride

Altitude ft / Distance miles

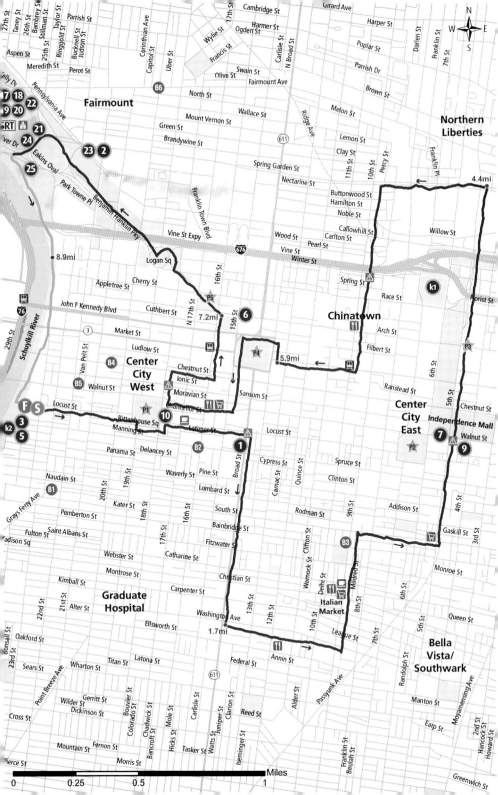

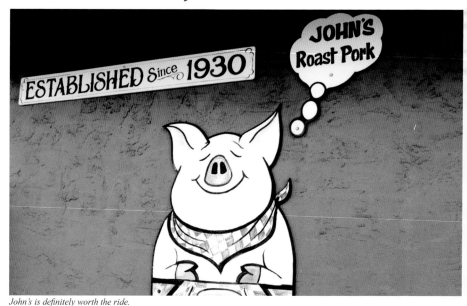

John's is definitely worth the ride.

At a Glance

Distance 3.0 miles   **Total Elevation** 47 feet

Terrain

The route features a few good bicycle lanes mixed in with your standard Philadelphia fare. It's a totally flat ride, and you will encounter the usual city obstacles such as broken glass and potholes.

Traffic

Traffic is heavy around Fourth and South, which also happen to be slightly narrower than some roads along the way. There's steady traffic on Moyamensing and Snyder, but you will have a hand with the bike lanes.

How to Get There

Both the 21 and 31 buses drop you directly at Penns Landing. You can also bike on over – Ride 1 will bring you close to the starting point on Front and Chestnut. There's also plenty of street parking in the area.

Food and Drink

This is obvious – you're going to want a cheesesteak or roast pork sandwich from John's. If for some confusing reason you do not want to try one of these delicious items, then you could stop at one of the many cafés along Fourth Street.

Side Trip

Jim's Steaks! There is always a line around the block. It's located at Fourth and South. Also, Tony Luke's is a little farther down Moyamensing on Snyder.

Links to ❶ ❷ ❻ ❼ ❽ ❿

Where to Bike Rating 🚲🚲🚲

About...

If you don't want to trek all the way out to Roxborough for a great steak (Ride 22: Cheesesteak Ride #2: Dalessandros), then try this short ride to John's Roast Pork in South Philly. It's just three miles from Old City, and it takes advantage of a few less traveled bicycle lanes including Moyamensing and Snyder.

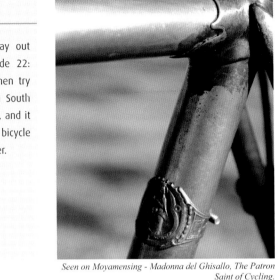

Seen on Moyamensing - Madonna del Ghisallo, The Patron Saint of Cycling.

A friend who lives in South Philly recently turned me onto the Moyamensing bicycle lanes as a way to bike down to his summer barbeques. As luck would have it, these lanes also bring you to Snyder Avenue, which drops you at the door (er, window?) of John's Roast Pork.

Here's a little known fact about John's: it actually won a James Beard award in 2006 in the "American Classics" category. It's been open since 1930, and the place is so delicious that you can only eat there Mon – Fri from 6:45am to 3:00pm (so plan your ride accordingly!). Believe it or not, there are one or two veggie options as well, and a slew of amazing breakfast sandwiches. You'll know you've arrived when you see the all too happy pig greeting you on Snyder Avenue.

But back to the ride: You'll start in Old City and head south. Walnut and Fourth Street can be busy and a little on the narrow side, so take your time here if you're new to street riding. The corner of Fourth and South can be particularly congested. It's also a great spot to consider getting your first tattoo.

Pedaling farther south, you'll ride through Southwark and Fabric Row. This is definitely one of my favorite streets in Philadelphia. Soak it all in! There is a lot to look at in the windows.

You'll cut over to Sixth via Catharine and then head farther south. Use caution around Sixth and Washington – Washington has faster traffic than other roads on this ride. There are bike lanes here, but they likely need a new coat of paint. The lanes end around Fourth, but you'll move into the right lane (separated from the main traffic on Washington Avenue), and turn down Moyamensing for more bicycle lanes.

The Moyamensing lanes also disappear from time to time, but you'll see plenty of bikers out here. The bus sometimes enjoys the bike lanes as well, so just be aware that you are likely to share some space with them as you travel through Pennsport. From Moyamensing, you'll make a left on Snyder and wait with baited breath until you reach the smiling pig! For a real cheesesteak challenge, take Center City Bike Lane Heaven (Ride 1) to Schuylkill Banks Park (Ride 3) to Cheesesteak Ride #2: Dalessandro's (Ride 22)! Don't forget some extra antacid.

Ride Log

0.0 Start at the park on Front and Chestnut St, and head south on Front St. You'll pass the back of the Ritz Theater.

0.1 Make a right onto Walnut St. Pedal into the Independence National Historical Park.

0.4 Take a left on Fourth St and pedal south.

0.8 Cross South St – Jim's is on the right if you can't wait for John's! Next you'll ride through Fabric Row and Southwark.

1.0 Right on Catharine St.

1.2 Left on Sixth St.

1.4 Left on Washington Ave. Watch for broken glass here! Pick up Washington Ave bike lanes.

1.6 The bike lanes end at Fourth St. Merge into the right lane, which is separated by a median from the main part of Washington.

1.7 Right on Moyamensing Ave bike lanes. You'll ride here for a while – continue to stay to the right.

2.2 Pass Dickinson Square Park to the right. You're in Pennsport!

2.6 Hang a left on Snyder Ave bike lanes.

3.0 Arrive at John's Roast Pork! After a sandwich, feel free to return the same way, but taking Fifth St north. You can also return via Columbus Blvd bicycle lanes if you are ready for a fast ride home.

P *P1* Ritz East, 125 South 2nd St
P2 Independence Hall
P3 Fabric Row
P4 Mummer's Museum, 1100 South 2nd St
P5 John's Roast Pork, 14 Snyder Ave

B *B1* Via Bicycle, 606 South 9th St
B2 Bicycle Revolutions, 756 s 4th St
B3 Performance Bicycle Shop, 1300 South Columbus Blvd, Riverview Plaza

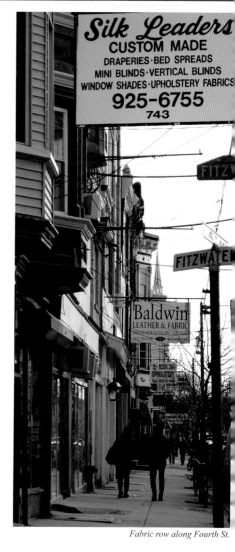

Fabric row along Fourth St.

Cheesesteak Ride #1: John's Roast Pork

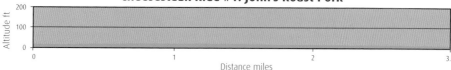

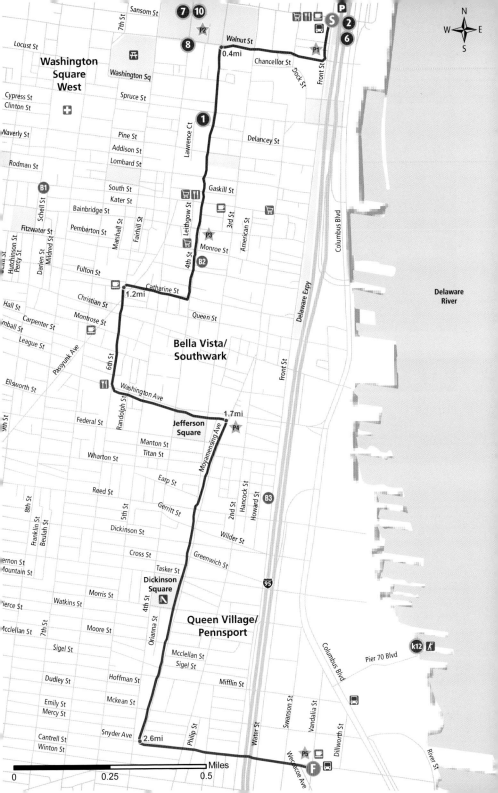

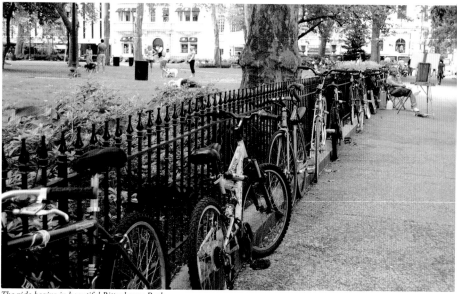

The ride begins in beautiful Rittenhouse Park.

At a Glance

Distance 7.3 miles   **Total Elevation** 101 feet

Terrain

You may find the road work, trolley tracks, and broken glass to be a hassle on your way to Frankford and Girard, or you may enjoy racing through the obstacle course that the city has so graciously laid out for you.

Traffic

You'll see steady traffic for most of the ride. There is significant traffic on Fifth Street and Girard, as well as the area around Logan Circle.

How to Get There

The ride begins in Rittenhouse Square, which is located on 18th and Walnut in Center City. If on bike, it's a short ride from the top of Schuylkill Banks Park (Ride 3). If coming from afar, your best bet is to hop on the train to Suburban station and make your way to Rittenhouse.

Food and Drink

There are places to stop on nearly every block of this route, with a number of great spots on Second and Third in Northern Liberties. Also, Johnny Brenda's has a pretty excellent menu.

Side Trip

This ride brings you direct to the Independence National Historical Park. So, if you want to check out the Constitution Center, Independence Hall, or the Independence Archeology Laboratory, then take Pine to Fifth, make a right on Fifth, and lock your bikes up before you hit the cobblestones!

Links to ❶ ❷ ❺ ❻ ❼ ❽ ❾

Where to Bike Rating

About...

This ride has so many fantastic details, including the Fifth Street tunnel, the bike lanes on Spring Garden and Pine, and one of my all time favorite roads in Philadelphia: 19th Street across Logan Circle. This fairly simple route will take you pretty far, but it has a "4" rating because you'll be pedaling alongside traffic for the duration of the ride.

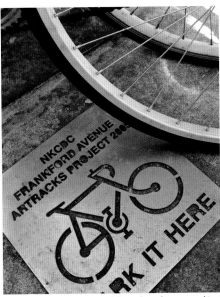

More bike parking than car parking!

Start off in glorious Rittenhouse Square, the largest greenspace in Center City and one of the best places in town for reading on a blanket, people-watching, and playing foursquare. From Rittenhouse, you'll hop on Locust and pedal east, making a right on 17th Street to pick up the Pine Street bicycle lanes.

After about 10 blocks on Pine, you'll shimmy up Seventh Street and ride a few blocks on Market on your way to the Fifth Street bicycle lanes. When on Market Street, please use caution and try to get in the left turning lane as soon as possible. Sure this appears to be a roundabout way to get to Fifth Street, but it's the best approach to avoid the grid of cobblestone streets in this part of town.

Once on Fifth, you're in for a delight – the traffic moves quickly but the bicycle lane gives you a good buffer. You'll hit the Fifth Street tunnel soon after the Constitution Center; it is very wide and there's a little downhill for added speed. You'll take Fifth to Spring Garden, and then Third Street up through Northern Liberties (there's a turn signal at the light) all the way up to Girard.

Take note: Girard has trolley tracks!! So be careful and see Ride 4 to learn how to conquer the tracks.

Johnny Brenda's is on the corner of Girard and Frankford, and it has a delicious menu of fresh local foods, a terrific beer list, and good shows too.

On your way home, you take Second Street through Northern Liberties, see a little more Spring Garden action, and then you'll be treated to 19th Street. You might not love this stretch as much as I do, what with its busses, narrow confines, bumpy portions and merging with Ben Franklin Parkway, but it sure is fun (especially late at night with little traffic). There's a slight downhill here, adding to the buzz. Stay to the right as you wind around Logan Circle, taking short advantage of the Ben Franklin bike lanes, and then peel off to pick up 19th Street again, which will take you back to Rittenhouse. Enjoy!

Ride Log

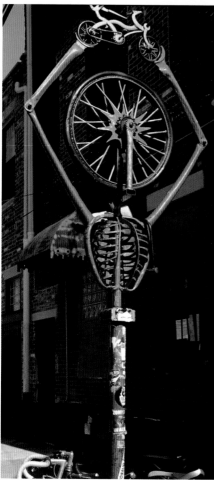

I love this little guy outside of JBs.

0.0 Begin at the southeast corner of Rittenhouse Park. Exit at 18th and Locust St. Take Locust east.

0.1 Right on 17th St.

0.3 Make a left on Pine to pick up those beautiful bike lanes.

0.6 Cross Broad St.

1.2 Make a left on Seventh St at the T-intersection. Go around Washington Square Park and bear right to continue on Seventh St.

1.4 Cross Walnut St.

1.7 Make a right on Market St – there's more traffic here, but it's just for a few blocks!

1.9 Left on Fifth St. There is a nice bike lane on Fifth St; follow it through the tunnel.

2.6 Right on Spring Garden to pick up bike lanes.

2.8 Get over to the left-hand lane. You'll make a left on Third St to pedal through Northern Liberties. Take Third to Girard.

3.4 Make a right on Girard and pedal to Frankford. Watch for the trolley tracks here!

3.8 JB's is on the corner of Girard and Frankford. After a sandwich or a dance party, head back down Girard towards Second St.

4.1 Left on Second St.

4.7 Right on Spring Garden bike lanes. Take this all the way across the city to 19th St.

6.2 Left on 19th St.

6.6 Bike around Logan Circle, continue down 19th St and take it all the way to the park.

7.3 Arrive back at Rittenhouse.

Center City to Johnny Brenda's

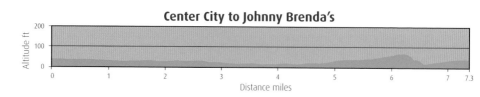

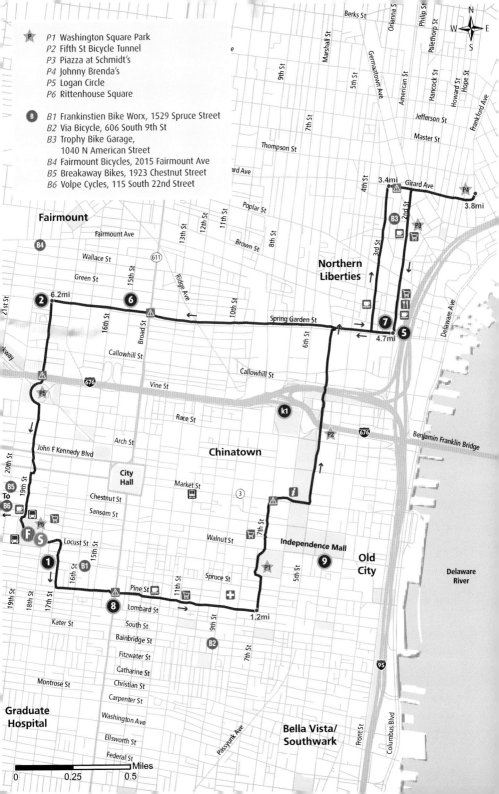

P1 Washington Square Park
P2 Fifth St Bicycle Tunnel
P3 Piazza at Schmidt's
P4 Johnny Brenda's
P5 Logan Circle
P6 Rittenhouse Square

B1 Frankinstien Bike Worx, 1529 Spruce Street
B2 Via Bicycle, 606 South 9th St
B3 Trophy Bike Garage,
    1040 N American Street
B4 Fairmount Bicycles, 2015 Fairmount Ave
B5 Breakaway Bikes, 1923 Chestnut Street
B6 Volpe Cycles, 115 South 22nd Street

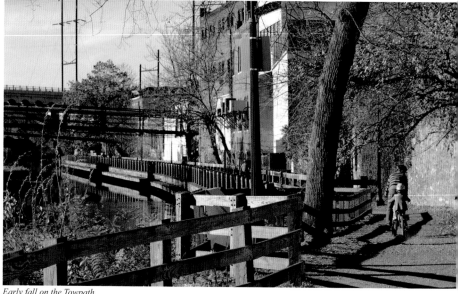

Early fall on the Towpath.

At a Glance

Distance 2.2 miles   **Total Elevation** 39 feet

Terrain

This towpath is a combination of boardwalk, dirt, and gravel, and it's as flat as the canal it follows.

Traffic

The Manayunk Towpath sees its share of folks walking, jogging, and cycling. Some portions are narrow and there are a few slight turns near bridges to navigate, so it is a good pick for a slow cycling jaunt.

How to Get There

The towpath runs in between Main Street and the Manayunk Canal. There is a very well marked entrance on the corner of Main and Lock streets. Buses 61 and 35 serve the area, but you can also take the Manayunk/Norristown line to the Manayunk train station. Of course the most fun way to get there is Ride 18: The Art Museum to Manayunk. It will drop you off at Lock Street.

Food and Drink

There are a million cafés on Main Street – no need to look far!

Side Trip

For a fun change of pace, streets that become promenades, live music, and artists from all over the country hanging out and selling their crafts, head to the annual Manayunk Arts Festival. It happens every June and is worth a peek.

Links to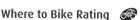

Where to Bike Rating

About...

At just four miles round trip the Manayunk Towpath provides a fun, leisurely trail for riders of all abilities. You'll pass a lot of families and little tykes here. The path also provides an off-road alternative to Main Street between the Kelly Drive and Valley Forge sections of the Schuylkill River Trail, but take note: the gravel towards the end of the path is best handled with fatter tires.

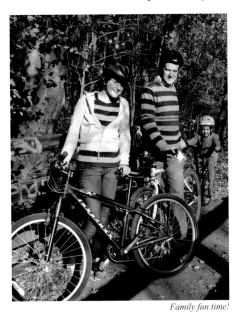

Family fun time!

The towpath is part of the Schuylkill River Heritage Area, which "celebrates the rich culture and history of the Schuylkill River watershed." It is designated as an important Industrial Revolution Site, for its role transporting goods at the turn of the 19th century. Many of the canal locks remain, as do the ruins of old textile mills. Signs about the history of the canal line the path – be sure to take the time to find out why this place is so special!

The trail, which runs between the canal and the back porches of some of the cafés on Main Street, becomes increasingly wooded as you pedal away from Lock Street. This is a great option for a family outing – you'll ride under a few dramatic bridges, and hopefully see lots of birds, fish and turtles mingling with the old industrial structures.

There are plenty of places to enter and exit the path along the way if you'd like a bite (for more information about what's happening in Manayunk, check out Ride 18). As the trail becomes more rugged, the gravel may prove nasty on your tires. Make sure to either bring a spare tube or plan to get pumped about a walk back to Cadence or Human Zoom for a fix.

The end of the towpath drops you off on Nixon Street, which is very close to the entrance to the Valley Forge section of the Schuylkill River Trail. Try it out if you'd like to extend your ride – this is a terrific bike path (see Ride 19: Schuylkill River Trail to Valley Forge for more information).

And here are a couple of things to look forward to: The Ivy Ridge Trail, which will stretch from the Ivy Ridge train station to the Manayunk station, and the Cynwyd Trail, which will connect Cynwyd station to the Manayunk viaduct, are both in the works. Visit www.completethetrail.org for updates. And, The Manayunk Development Corporation is organizing a total restoration of the canal locks.

Ride Log

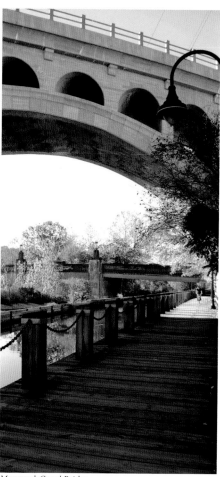

This ride log is super easy – just grab your bicycle and hop on the trail at Main and Lock streets.

0.2 Pass Cotton St entrance.

0.4 Ride under the Green Ln bridge.

0.7 Pass Leverington Ave – this area is known as the Riparian Slope Forest.

0.9 Ride under the Fountain St bridge. Check out all those vines!

1.0 For the next mile, the trail becomes a bit more rugged with large gravel and a tree root here and there. The path will also have more and more shade trees.

2.2 Turn around and head back to Lock St, or if you want to ride a little bit farther, exit the towpath and follow Nixon St to the Valley Forge section of the SRT (Ride 19).

P1 Venice Island Recreation Center
P2 Manayunk Wall

B1 Cadence Performance Cycling,
4323 Main Street
BR1 Human Zoom, 4159 Main Street

Manayunk Canal Bridge.

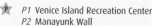

Manayunk Towpath

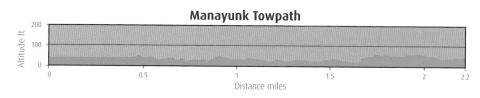

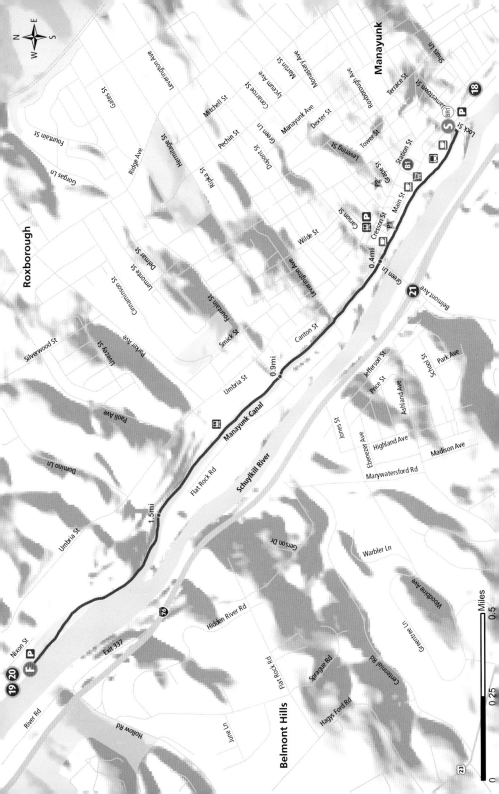

Forbidden Drive

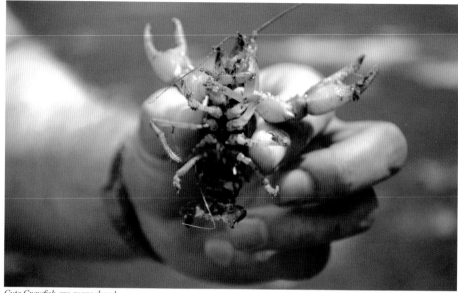

Cute Crawfish are everywhere!

At a Glance

Distance 13.2 miles   **Total Elevation** 146 feet

Terrain

Forbidden Drive is a timeless gravel path along the Wissahickon Creek in lush Fairmount Park.

Traffic

Oh lots! Runners, hikers, frogs, and cyclists all enjoy this wooded area.

How to Get There

There are two main entrances to Forbidden Drive; one is located on Ridge Avenue across from the Kelly Drive portion of the Schuylkill River Trail, and the other at trail's end just off Northwestern Avenue in Chestnut Hill which has a large parking lot. Buses 1, 9, and 27 will drop you near the Ridge Avenue entrance, though you could also bike down from Boathouse Row (Ride 17).

Food and Drink

You'll pass the Valley Green Inn, rumored to have been in business since 1683. The inn offers a lovely oasis by the creek to stop and have a cold drink or a longer gourmet lunch. Bruno's (Ride 20), a comfortable diner, is near the northwestern entrance.

Side Trip

Devil's Pool is just off Forbidden Drive, near Livezey Lane. Thanks to recent cleanup efforts by The Friends of the Wissahickon, the shallow swimming hole is coming back to life as an adventurous spot to cool off in the summer.

Links to (18) (19) (20) (21) (22) (30)

Where to Bike Rating

About...

The shaded Forbidden Drive, which runs along the Wissahickon Creek, is a favorite for cyclists and runners to escape the sounds of the city. The rumblings of the creek offer a delightful contrast to the daily beeps and horns of downtown, plus, there are lots of critters roaming around the drive. Nature in the city comes in all shapes and sizes, including that baby crawfish. We'll take it. It's packed gravel, so best to bring your fat tires.

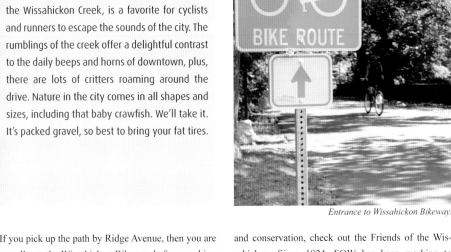

Entrance to Wissahickon Bikeway.

If you pick up the path by Ridge Avenue, then you are actually on the Wissahickon Bikeway before reaching Forbidden Drive proper. The bikeway was revamped in 2007 to improve the connection between the Wissahickon and Kelly Drive. It offers cyclists a 1.5 mile paved path that runs through Fairmount Park alongside Lincoln Drive.

Once you reach Forbidden Drive, the trail becomes packed gravel. There are a lot of arched bridges along the way, and one red covered bridge that juts out of the greenery in a striking color contrast worthy of the brightest oil paints. Stop by the creek and dunk your feet or touch the water with your hands – you may catch yourself a cute little crawfish!

The Valley Green Inn stands serenely at the midpoint of the ride. Built on land purchased from William Penn in 1685, the inn has a long meandering history. T.A. Daily wrote in 1922 that, "The charm of Valley Green varies not only with the seasons, but with the day of the week and the hour of the day." Reminiscent of a different time and place, the benches across from the inn offer the perfect spot to take a break from the ride and sit by the creek.

For more information about park activities, events, and conservation, check out the Friends of the Wissahickon. Since 1924, FOW has been working to "preserve the natural beauty and wildness of the Wissahickon Valley and stimulate public interest therein." They also have lots of volunteer opportunities.

When you reach Northwestern Avenue, make a right on road to reach Bruno's, Chestnut Hill College, or continue down the hill to reach the entrance to Morris Arboretum. Or just have a rest and turn back towards the city!

It's pretty hard to get lost on Forbidden Drive! Just follow the path.

Ride Log

0.0 Cross Ridge Ave at the entrance to the Wissahickon Bike Trail. Follow the signs and hop on the trail!

1.0 Cross the bridge over the Wissahickon Creek.

1.2 You'll come to an intersection. Make a left here, and pedal through a small area before entering Forbidden Dr. Continue along Forbidden Dr (packed gravel). You'll stay on this trail for the remainder of the ride.

3.7 Devil's Pool will be on your right, just off Livezey Ln.

4.0 Come to the Valley Green Inn, on your left.

5.5 The beautiful red covered bridge will be on your right. Continue past this bridge.

6.1 Cross Bells Mills Rd.

6.6 You'll reach the trailhead of Forbidden Dr. When you're ready to head home, turn around and…

7.0 Cross Bells Mill Rd.

7.7 Red covered bridge.

9.1 Pass Valley Green Inn.

12.0 Cross the small parking area, and make a right to pick up the Wissahickon Bikeway.

13.2 Back at the Ridge Ave entrance!

P1 Valley Green Inn
P2 Thomas Mill Covered Bridge
P3 Morris Arboretum

B1 Cadence Performance Cycling,
    4323 Main Street
B2 Human Zoom, 4159 Main Street
B3 Wissahickon Cyclery,
    7837 Germantown Avenue
B4 Philly Electric Wheels
    7102 Germantown Avenue

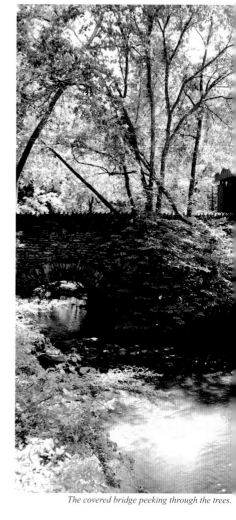

The covered bridge peeking through the trees.

Forbidden Drive

Altitude ft

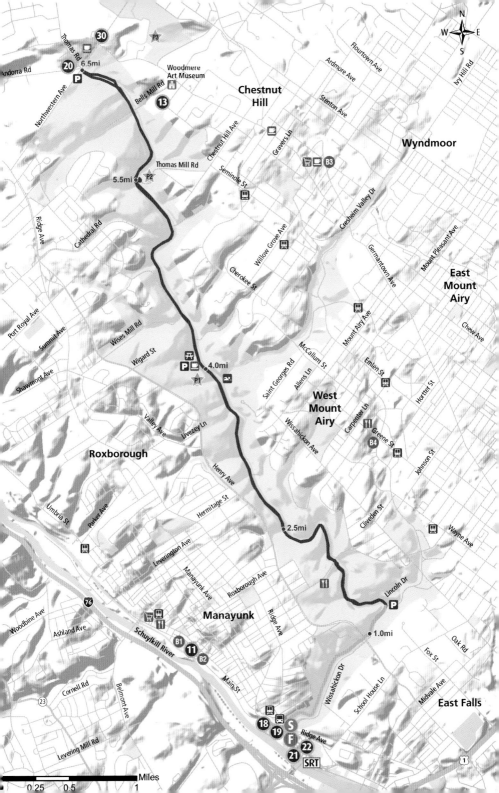

Linda's Chestnut Hill Loop

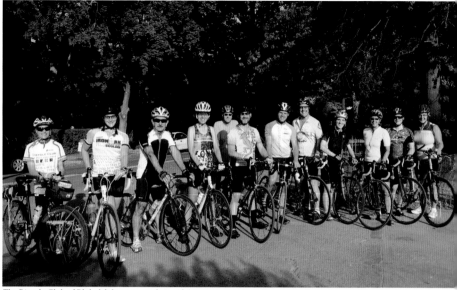

The Bicycle Club of Philadelphia gets ready to ride!

At a Glance

Distance 13.6 miles   **Total Elevation** 456 feet

Terrain

This log includes a mix of residential and city streets, with a couple of steep hills.

Traffic

The traffic here is pretty relaxed, save for a few spots around busy intersections (including Germantown Avenue, Lincoln Drive, and Bells Mill Road). But you'll be in good company - there are a ton of cyclists in this part of town.

How to Get There

Take the train to the Chestnut Hill West line to Allens Lane – the ride starts here on the corner of Nippon and West Allens Lane. Easy peasy.

Food and Drink

Weaver's Way Coop is the place to be! It's on Carpenters Lane in Mount Airy. Of course, there are also many spots on Germantown Avenue for a snack.

Side Trip

Take Bethlehem Pike all the way to Germantown Avenue and lock up your bikes for a stroll through Chestnut Hill. This is a fun area of the city; the sidewalks are lined with trees, cafes, and shops. You'll be at the "top of the hill" – walk down a ways to find Bredenbeck's Bakery and Ice Cream, just after Harwell Lane.

Links to

Where to Bike Rating

About...

Thank you to Linda McGrane, President of the Bicycle Club of Philadelphia (BCP), for this fun, meandering loop through Chestnut Hill and Mount Airy. Linda knows all the best roads in the city, and this is a beautiful area for bicycling – there are a lot of shady green trees, and many of the streets are well paved and extra wide. The loop has a few turns that double back, a couple of steep hills, and one very enjoyable downhill.

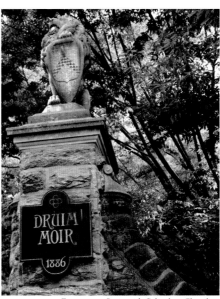

Entrance to Springside School on Cherokee.

Chestnut Hill, once a vacation spot for wealthy city dwellers, is now a beautiful residential area that feels like a suburb even though it is technically within the city of Philadelphia – many of the homes here will have you oooing and aaaahing! It is especially beautiful in the spring and summer, when all of the trees and gardens are blossoming.

The ride starts conveniently at the Allens Lane train station, a popular meeting place for BCP group rides. You'll start off exploring a little bit of Mount Airy before making your way into Chestnut Hill. You'll travel to and fro on some of the same roads, including McCallum Street, Mermaid Lane, and Willow Grove Avenue.

Traffic will be easy for the most part, but a few streets, including Cresheim Valley Drive and Willow Grove Avenue, will have heavy car traffic. Please be careful around a few tricky intersections, including Lincoln Drive, Germantown Avenue, and Bells Mill Road. And some fun: Germantown Avenue is cobblestones!

The bend in Cherokee before it becomes West Harwell Lane is blind. There's a downhill here, so enjoy it and get your speed up but be sure to stay to the right.

After the turn you'll be greeted by a very stately site – the back of the Philadelphia Cricket Club, founded in 1854. If you tire early, you can hitch a ride back to the city at the St. Martins train station, which is just ahead.

Soon, you'll be in the heart of Chestnut Hill. The roads are much quieter here, and the lack of cars, surprise hills and strange curves make for great riding.

You may notice this map has a lot of little loops and double backs (read: totally illogical!). This is not a ride about getting somewhere fast; it's a ride about wandering through a lovely neighborhood just to see what's around the corner. So take your time and enjoy yourself.

If you like riding around here, check out Ride 20: Boathouse Row to Bruno's. For more information about BCP group rides, a great way to get to know the city on a bike, check out their website: www.phillybikeclub.org.

Ride 13 - Linda's Chestnut Hill Loop

Ride Log

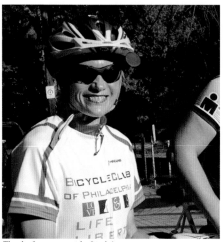

Thanks for a great ride, Linda!

0.0 Start at the Allens Ln train station; make a left on Nippon St.

0.1 Right on Bryan St.

0.3 Right of West Mt Pleasant Ave.

0.4 Left on Mower St.

0.5 Right on West Sedgwick St.

0.6 Left on Cresheim Rd.

0.8 Right on Carpenter Ln and follow for a ways (you'll have to cross Lincoln Dr – sorry!).

1.5 Right on Sherman, which becomes North Mt Pleasant Rd.

1.9 Left on McCallum St – a very well traveled road for bicycles.

2.4 Cross the McCallum St bridge.

2.6 Right on Mermaid Ln.

3.1 Left on St. Martins Ln.

3.3 Right on Springfield Ave.

3.4 Right on Cresheim Rd (fun downhill!).

3.6 Right on Lincoln Dr, but just for a bit!

3.65 Left on Cresheim Valley Dr.

4.3 Left on Crittenden St (if you hit Stenton, you've gone too far).

4.7 Left on Willow Grove Ave.

6.0 Right on Cherokee St. Follow Cherokee down the hill and around the bend; it becomes West Hartwell Ln.

6.6 Right on St. Martins Ln.

6.8 A left back onto Willow Grove Ave.

6.9 Quick left on Seminole St.

7.3 Left on Gravers Ln.

7.4 Right back onto St. Martins Ln.

7.5 Left onto Seminole St.

7.8 Right on W Chestnut Hill Ave.

8.0 Left on Crefeld St.

8.6 Right on West Hampton Rd – you'll be heading downhill for a bit here!

8.8 Left on Green Tree Rd.

8.9 Quick Right on East Bells Mill Rd.

9.3 Right on Stenton Ave/Bethlehem Pike; follow Bethlehem uphill.

10.0 Hairpin turn onto Summit St, just before Germantown Ave.

10.3 Right on Prospect Ave.

10.5 Right on East Gravers Ln, then a quick left on Crittenden St.

10.9 Left back onto your favorite – Willow Grove Ave!

11.8 Left on St. Martins Ln.

12.0 Right on Mermaid Ln.

12.5 Left on McCallum St.

13.0 Left on West Allens Ln.

13.6 Right on Cresheim Rd and back to the station.

Linda's Chestnut Hill Loop

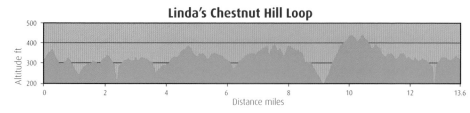

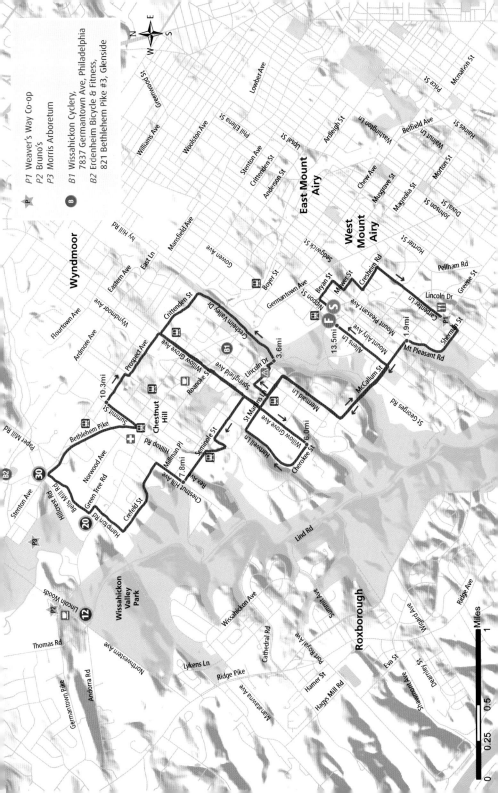

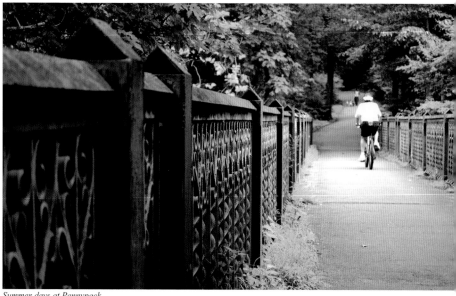

Summary days at Pennypack.

At a Glance

Distance 15.2 miles **Total Elevation** 122 feet

Terrain

Pennypack offers cyclists a long, paved path through the woods – in Northeast Philadelphia! You'll enjoy a mix of short hills and flat riding along the creek. There are also gravel mountain bike trails off the main path.

Traffic

This is a mixed use trail, and there is steady traffic from the bicycling and jogging set in warmer months. Horseback riding is also popular on the gravel trails.

How to Get There

Pennypack is located in Northeast Philadelphia. There is ample parking at the trail head off Shady Lane. The 67 bus will drop you at Verree Road and Tustin Street, and the 58 at Bustleton and Winchester Avenue – both a stone's throw from trail entrances.

Food and Drink

Bring a picnic! If you forget, there's usually a sandwich stand by the Shady Lane entrance with cold drinks. If you're starving and looking for an on-road biking adventure, Sweet Lucy's has delicious barbeque. It's past Frankford on State Road.

Side Trip

Pennypack Park hosts an outdoor concert series on Wednesday evenings in the summer. Throw a lawn chair on your rack and bike on down! You can check out the schedule online at www.pennypackpark.com.

Links to 30

Where to Bike Rating

About...

Pennypack Park is one of a kind in Philadelphia. No other paved bicycling trail in the city is as long or as secluded. The path follows the curves of the Pennypack Creek, an area that was originally preserved for its ornithological diversity. While you will pedal under enormous bridges and hear the whir of major thruways – Route 1, Bustleton, and Rhawn, to name a few –the park still has quiet pockets that will help you forget it's smack in the middle of the city.

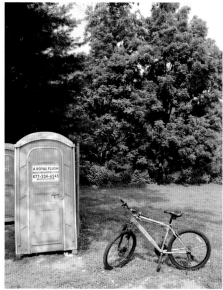

Potty break.

Welcome to Pennypack Park! This shady path offers city dwellers a lovely change of pace. Because it is straight and hilly, Pennypack makes for a great exercise or training route – you won't need to fumble with any cue sheets here. This is a popular place for cyclists and runners on the weekends and after work – head over in the mornings to have the trail to yourself and the deer!

Pennypack is also perfect for families and lazy Sunday afternoon rides. The park itself is about 1600 acres of woodlands, offering an oasis in Northeast Philadelphia. Historic structures and stone bridges pop up along the main trail (the park celebrated its 100th Anniversary in 2005), and gravel paths lead off into the woods. The top half (from Shady Lane to Bustleton) was short, fun spikes every half mile or so, while the bottom half (Bustleton to Frankford) is much flatter. The trail is very curvy, and there are a few blind spots, so be sure to ride slowly if you can't see what's coming straight ahead. Like me you could be surprised by one of the many deer who didn't hear the chimes of my little bicycle bell!

The riding log for this trail is very simple – Pennypack is just one long path that runs from Shady Lane

in Fox Chase all the way to State Road in Holmesburg. There are points to pick up the path at all of the major intersections, and bicycle traffic runs fluidly in each direction. I chose to turn around at Frankford Avenue for a 15 mile round trip, but you may want to explore farther.

If you want to learn more about the history and ecology of Pennypack, you may want to stop in on the Pennypack Environmental Center on Verree Road. They host an open house on the first Saturday of every month, with exhibits, a small public library, bird watches, and a picnic area.

For the naturalist/bike enthusiast, hop on the Fairmount Park website to grab "The Birds of Pennypack Park" brochure. It outlines all of the bird life you may encounter, along with their relative abundance and season. Pennypackpark.org also has a selection of "Noteworthy" trees along the path.

However you choose to experience Pennypack, it's worth a go!

Ride Log

0.0 Pick up the north end of the trail by the Shady Ln entrance.

0.7 Cross Verree Rd. The Pennypack Environmental Center is just before Verree.

2.4 Cross Krewstown Rd.

3.2 Ride by Bustleton Ave. You'll go up a steep hill next.

3.5 Pop out on Winchester Ave and duck back into the woods.

4.1 Ride under Rt 1.

4.8 Cross Holme Ave.

5.2 Cross Rhawn St and follow the curves.

6.0 Cross Rhawn again.

6.3 Entering an open area here – the concert stage is coming up on your left.

6.5 Cross Welsh Rd.

7.6 Hit Frankford Ave. If you wish, you can cross Frankford and pick up the trail a little ways farther to State Rd. But if you haven't yet, Frankford is as good a place to turn around as any.

9.1 Cross Rhawn one more time.

12.0 Cross back over Bustleton.

14.4 Bike by Verree Rd.

15.2 And back to the beginning!

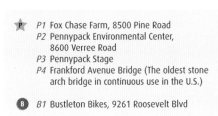

P1 Fox Chase Farm, 8500 Pine Road
P2 Pennypack Environmental Center, 8600 Verree Road
P3 Pennypack Stage
P4 Frankford Avenue Bridge (The oldest stone arch bridge in continuous use in the U.S.)

B1 Bustleton Bikes, 9261 Roosevelt Blvd

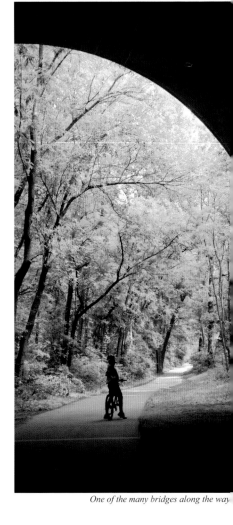

One of the many bridges along the way

Pennypack Park

Altitude ft

Distance miles

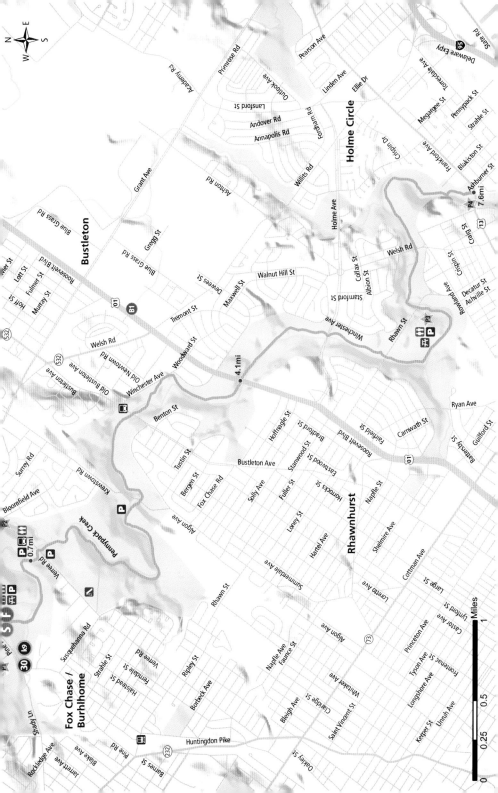

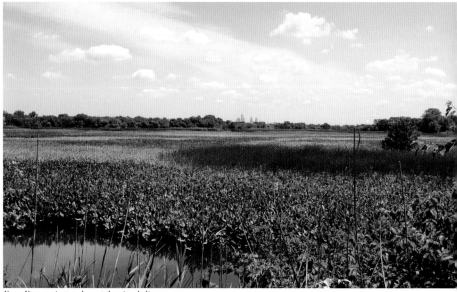

Yes... You can just make out the city skyline.

At a Glance

Distance 6.6 miles   **Total Elevation** 24 feet

Terrain

John Heinz is a flat packed gravel path through wooded areas and tidal marshes. One section, the nature path, is a tight singletrack.

Traffic

John Heinz is a well kept secret. The trails have their fair share of birds chirping and insects humming, but they are often on the quiet side in terms of humans.

How to Get There

You'll find parking at the 86th Street and Lindberg Boulevard entrance. The 37 and 108 buses will drop you off at 84th and Lindberg Avenue. You can also take regional rail to Eastwick station – this stop is a couple of blocks south east of the refuge entrance.

Food and Drink

There isn't much in the way of food and drink here, so best to bring extra fluids and a picnic lunch. There are water fountains at the trail head.

Side Trip

The Cusano Environmental Education Center is located near the trail head. The center's distinctive mission is to "demonstrate, within an urban setting, the importance of the natural world to the human quality of life and inspire visitors to become responsible stewards of the environment." They offer loads of trail information and specie checklists. You can also rent fishing rods!

Where to Bike Rating

About...

There are few places in Philadelphia where one can be surrounded by nature long enough to dismiss the stresses of the city. The John Heinz Refuge, which circles Tinicum Marsh, offers visitors this opportunity. Nature enthusiasts and birders will love the refuge – over 280 species have been recorded here. You may want to bring a pair of more rugged tires for this outing; the gravel trails referee an epic game of hide and seek between old tree roots and big rocks.

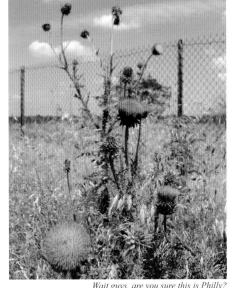

Wait guys, are you sure this is Philly?

The U.S. Fish and Wildlife Service maintain the John Heinz trails, which total about 10 miles. You should feel free to explore as many as you wish – they all head back to the entrance sooner or later. The map shows the main route through the park and access to the nature path, but there is also a loop around the large body of water known as the impoundment.

You'll see an unexpected array of wildlife in the refuge, including turtles, frogs, butterflies, deer, rabbits and gophers. But the big draw to John Heinz is the variety of bird species in the area, including the Bald Eagle and the Great Blue Heron. The refuge posts an updated list of specie sightings and relative abundance to their website fairly regularly.

The path itself is mostly packed gravel, winding through a couple of tree covered turns. The foliage is lush in the summer, with lots of animals and birds hiding in the leaves. The boardwalk near the entrance offers a nice spot to watch for fish and turtles.

Some of the sights indicating that you are, in fact, still in the city include visions of the Sunoco oil refinery peeking through the trees over Darby Creek, and farther on, the stretch of trail that runs alongside I-95. And, of course, who could forget the hundreds of airplanes that take off from PHL International right around the corner? But it's all part of the quirky experience of nature in the city.

At mile 3.1 there is a little bridge that leads to the nature path. If you are a beginner rider, lock your bikes to the bridge and try taking a romp through the woods for a change of pace. More expert riders will enjoy the singletrack (which has some tree root and foxholes). The path is quite narrow. You have to watch out for poison ivy and stinging nettle along the way, but this trail is really the place that makes you forget you are in the middle of the city. It hooks up with the packed gravel trail and eventually loops around.

Ride Log

 P1 Cusano Environmental Education Center,
86th St and Lindberg Blvd
P2 Philadelphia International Airport

0.0 Pick up the trail near the entrance to the refuge on Lindberg Ave. Head southwest on the wide gravel packed road. You'll see Darby Creek to the right.
Pass the boardwalk over the impoundment to the left (a great place to stop and watch wildlife).

1.4 The road forks here, and each path leads to the same trail in roughly the same distance. Make a left and enjoy the shaded path.

1.7 Go right when you hit the packed gravel road alongside I-95. Yes, it is funny to see the highway. Now you've experienced an urban wildlife refuge!

2.1 Continue along this trail.

3.1 The red bridge will lead you to the nature path. It is a narrow singletrack perched on a 15ft wide stretch of land splitting the tidal marshes. If you are a confident rider and choose to pedal through, it will drop you off at the 2.1 mile junction. If you just want to check it out on foot, lock your bike to the bridge and walk on in!

4.5 Assuming you pedaled through, you'll find yourself at the familiar 2.1 mile junction. If you left your bikes, you'll have to backtrack along either the nature path or the I-95 route to pick them up.

4.6 Continue along funny I-95 trail.

4.9 Continue past this familiar spot (marker 1.7) to make a giant loop, or take a left to head back the way you came.

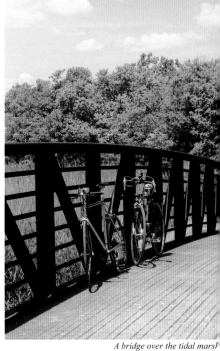

A bridge over the tidal marsh

5.9 Assuming you took the long way, pedal left to follow the bend in the trail.

6.4 This is an excellent bird and wildlife observation area. The boardwalk is nearby as well, in case you want to see more!

6.6 Trail pops out at the entrance to the refuge.

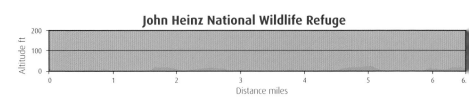

John Heinz National Wildlife Refuge

Altitude ft

200

100

0

0   1   2   3   4   5   6   6.

Distance miles

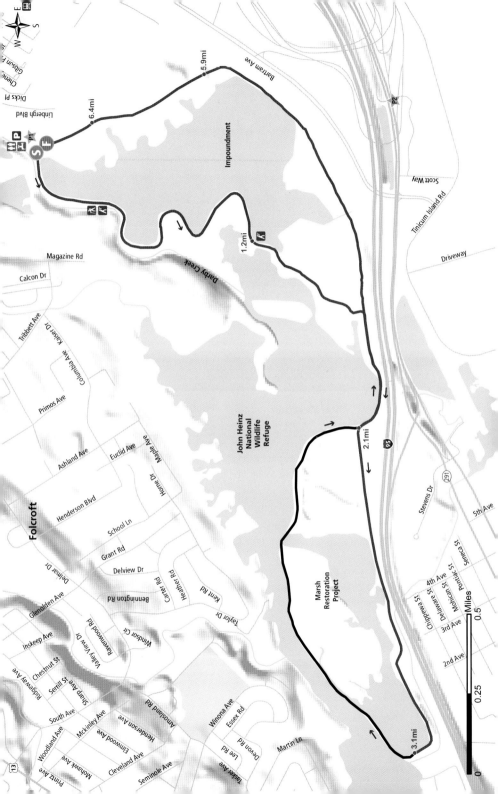

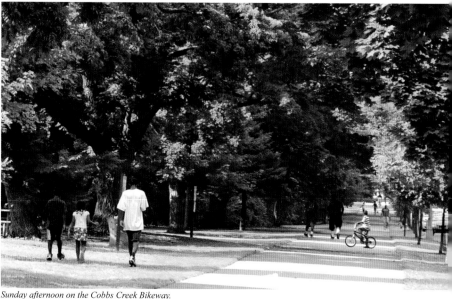

Sunday afternoon on the Cobbs Creek Bikeway.

At a Glance

Distance 7.0 miles   **Total Elevation** 107 feet

Terrain

A multi-use paved path that runs along the road, except for a small section that winds through the woods. As with many other routes in Philadelphia, be on the lookout for scattered glass and light debris patiently waiting atop the pavement to pop your new tires.

Traffic

The Cobbs Creek Bikeway generally has less foot and bicycle traffic than the paths nearer to Center City, but the picnic areas, basketball courts and playgrounds along the way are hopping in the warmer months.

How to Get There

You'll find a parking lot near the northern end of the path on 63rd and Walnut Street in West Philadelphia. The Spruce Street bike lanes and the 21 bus will also get you close by.

Food and Drink

Not many options along Cobbs Creek, so best to brin some snacks and extra water for your ride.

Side Trip

Check out *Love Letter*, a collection of 50 rooftop mu rals by former graffiti artist Steve Powers for the Mura Arts Program. This awesome collection of public a runs along Market Street between 45th and 63rd. The Market/Frankford El gives a great view.

Links to

As of February 2010, funding had been secured t build the 1.5 mile 58th Street Connector, which wi link to Bartram's Garden (Ride 24).

Where to Bike Rating

About...

Far out in West Philadelphia you'll find the Cobbs Creek Bikeway, a quiet path that stretches from 63rd Street and Market on down to 70th. City and nature collide along this ride – to one side you'll see the creek and its verdant trees, to the other you'll watch the cityscape of West Philly fly by. This juxtaposition makes for some of the most unique urban riding that Philadelphia has to offer.

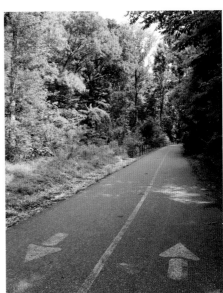

Around the switchback.

Starting out at the northern tip of the recreation path, you'll pass the Laura Sims Skate House and the Cobbs Creek Recreation Center. The pool by the rec center is barely visible from the path, but the giggling and splashing can be heard all the way down the block in the summer months.

The Cobbs Creek Community Environmental Education Center is up next. CCCEEC is housed in a beautifully restored stable on 63rd and Catharine. It offers programming for activists of all ages, from the Senior Environmental Corps to The Park Management for Youth Program.

The path follows the rhythm of the city blocks, and in some sections you'll have to cross the street in order to reach the path on the next block. On 61st Street (seems illogical but the street number is correct, it's just a funny angle) the path curves to the right around Cobbs Creek Park. You'll continue along path adjacent to the park until reaching Baltimore Avenue. After crossing Baltimore, follow the path past the basketball courts to enter the woods.

This section of the path is quieter than the others. You'll pass an old railroad trestle sprouting up from the ground, a striking sight in the summer when surrounded by big bushy tree leaves. It looks like the top of the canopy. Continue along the path and follow the creek before hitting a steep switchback – the only hill of the ride.

When you emerge from the woods, you'll be riding alongside the curvy Cobbs Creek Parkway. The old stone walls after Mount Moriah Cemetery seem to hold the stories of centuries. This is my favorite section of the path. You'll pass under a few scattered bridges before you are jolted out of your escape by busy 70th Street, marking the end of the path.

After you turn around at 70th Street to head back north, you may feel something of a slow burn – there will be a slight incline for most of the way back to 63rd Street.

Ride Log

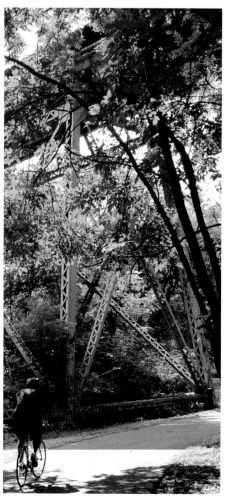

That really cool old railway trestle.

0.0 Start on Walnut St heading south on the Cobbs Creek Bikeway. Pass the Laura Sims Skate House and the Cobbs Creek Recreation Center to the right.

0.6 Pass the Cobbs Creek Environmental Education Center at 63rd and Catharine.

1.1 Make a right at 61st St to follow the path around Cobbs Creek Park.

1.3 Cross Baltimore Ave and follow the path into the woods.

1.5 Pass under the railroad trestle.

1.6 Follow the switchback and enjoy the climb!

1.7 Pop out on 59th St and make a right to continue along the path.

2.5 Pass Mt. Moriah Cemetery to the right.

3.3 Ride underneath the 65th St bridge.

3.5 Reach 70th St. Turn around and head north back towards 63rd and Walnut.

7.0 Back at Walnut and ride's end.

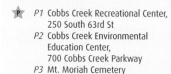

P1 Cobbs Creek Recreational Center,
   250 South 63rd St
P2 Cobbs Creek Environmental
   Education Center,
   700 Cobbs Creek Parkway
P3 Mt. Moriah Cemetery

B1 Swaray's Bike Shop, 612 52nd St
B2 Firehouse Bicycles, 701 South 50th St

The Cobbs Creek Bikeway

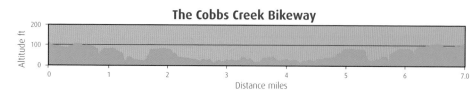

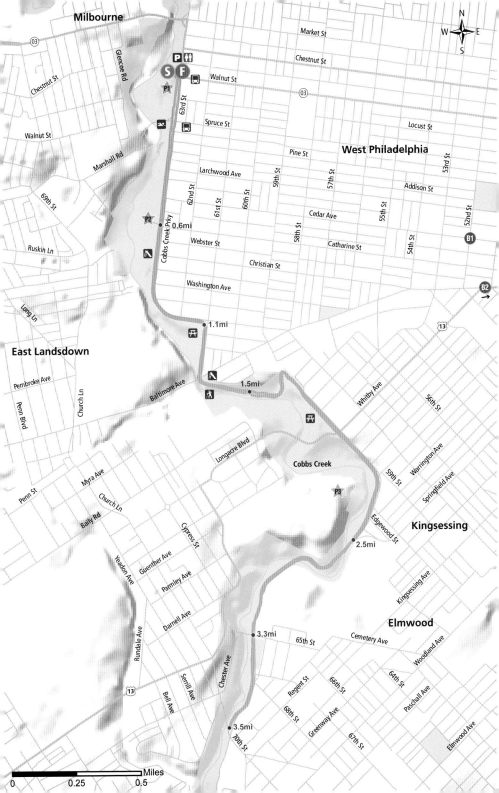

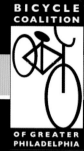

Do **you** bike Philly?

Join the Bicycle Coalition of Greater Philadelphia!

BICYCLE COALITION OF GREATER PHILADELPHIA

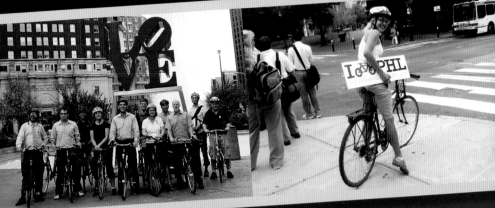

Your membership supports:

- The work of our eight local advocacy committees.

- Our Bicycle Ambassadors program - Bicycle Ambassadors encourage adult bicyclists to ride more often and more safely as well as educate motorists on the rules of the road and provide tips for sharing the road.

- Philadelphia's new bike plan, a blueprint for Mayor Nutter's goal of creating the "Greenest City in America".

- Philadelphia's Bike Month in May with events like Bike to Work Day and the Commuter Challenge.

- Our campaign to have Pennsylvania, New Jersey and Delaware adopt statewide complete streets policies to ensure bicyclists are planned for in all road and transportation projects.

- The Delaware Valley's presence at the National Bike Summit to make sure biking is an important part of next year's federal transportation bill.

- Bringing bike sharing to Philadelphia.

- Expanding Bike Philly's car-free route.

Visit us online today!

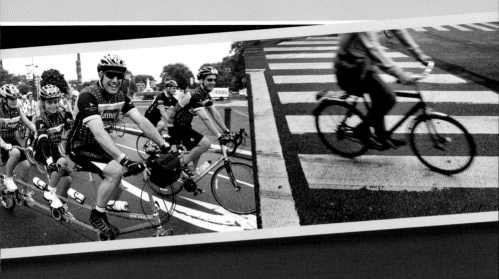

We cannot make any of our plans come true without the support of our members. Many of our members choose to give a dollar a week to make their ride better. Committing to a dollar a week is a strong step towards making the Delaware Valley a more bicycle-friendly community — and it costs less than what you spend on gas or SEPTA – or even coffee!

Membership benefits include:

- The monthly CycleGram e-newsletter.
- Discounts at over 30 bike shops and other companies in the region.
- Discounted registration at Bike Philly and Bike Freedom Valley.
- An invitation to our annual meeting.
- Your membership dues are tax deductible.

Most important of all, you will get the satisfaction of supporting better biking. Your support of the Bicycle Coalition will help you – and your neighbors – find more ways to bike for exercise, recreation and commuting.

Join today by calling **(215) 242-9253** or visiting us on the web at **www.bicyclecoalition.org**

www.bicyclecoalition.org

Art Museum Departures

A Philadelphia tradition, the Art Museum is a major meeting place for cyclists who want to head out of the city for an afternoon.

Its massive popularity comes from its position on the Schuylkill River Trail (SRT), a network of multi-use trails in Southeastern Pennsylvania. When completed, the trail is projected to total almost 130 miles!

All the old standards are all here – Philadelphia to Manayunk (Ride 18), SRT to Valley Forge (Ride 19), and Center City to Bruno's in Chestnut Hill (Ride 20). But you'll also find routes that give a tour of West Fairmount Park, guide you through the Mainline, and bring you all the way out to Bartram's Garden.

And now for the great news – In the summer Martin Luther King Jr Drive (West River Drive) is closed to traffic on weekends. Head out here for familiar faces, tons of extra space, and perfectly paved car free miles to add to your route.

A side note: many of the Philadelphia cycling clubs meet at the Art Museum. If you're looking for the Italian Fountain meeting spot, it is right there in between Lloyd Hall (1 Boathouse Row) and the back of the Art Museum.

So whether you're out for a lazy Sunday afternoon ride around the loop or racing from Philly to Valley Forge, you'll find an idea for a ride you've never taken before in this chapter. And we've placed an SRT icon on every map where the Schuylkill River Trail links up to a ride, so just look for the SRT icon, and you'll never be far from home!

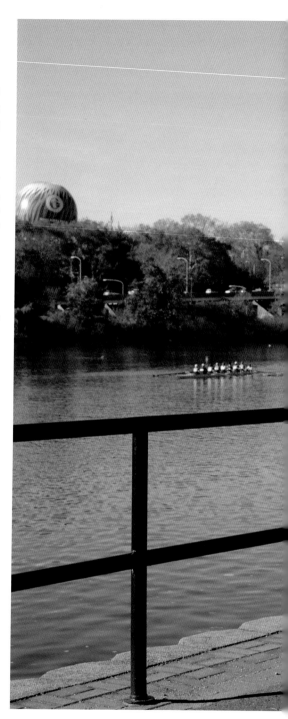

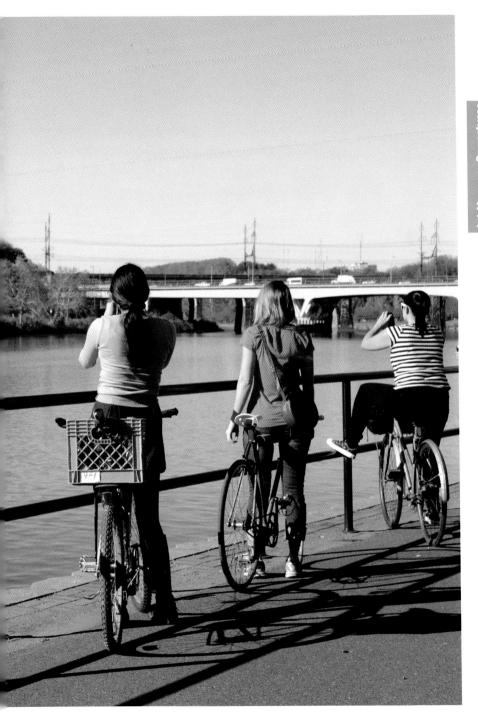

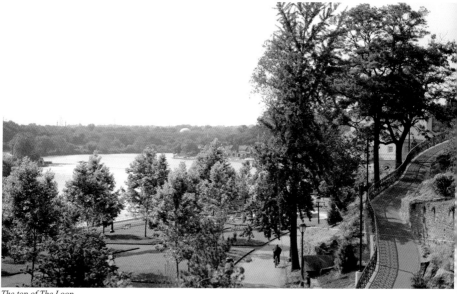

The top of The Loop.

At a Glance

Distance 8.2 miles   **Total Elevation** 56 feet

Terrain

The Loop is a paved mixed-use recreation path that loops around the Schuylkill River.

Traffic

The Loop is one of the most popular destinations for outdoor activities in Philadelphia, and it attracts the lion's share of city cyclists and runners. The stretch near boathouse row always has the heaviest traffic – best to take it slow until you pass the Viking statue.

How to Get There

The log begins at Lloyd Hall on Kelly Drive. Septa bus routes 7, 32, 38, 43 and 48 serve the museum area. If driving, you'll find ample parking behind the Art Museum and Boathouse Row.

Food and Drink

From noon to dusk you'll pass Chief, the nice old guy who stocks soft pretzels, pinwheels, and cold drinks at the stand across from The University Barge Club on Boathouse Row. The bench across from the stand is dedicated to Chief – he's been in this spot since 1946!

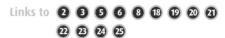

Where to Bike Rating

About...

The Loop, referred to as such because it is by far the most popular spot for cycling in Philadelphia, needs little introduction. The path that winds along the Schuylkill River includes stunning views of Boathouse Row, the old waterworks, and bridge after bridge over the water. Martin Luther King Jr. Drive (formerly West River Drive) is closed to traffic most weekends April – October, giving folks plenty of extra room to pedal in the summer.

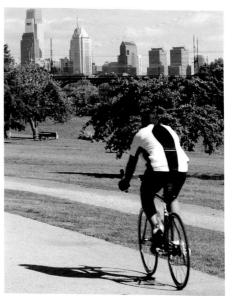

Biking near the Angels statue.

The ride log starts behind the Art Museum where the Schuylkill River Trail meets the Schuylkill Banks Park, but you can pick up the path at nearly any point along the way. The stretch between the Art Museum and Boathouse Row will be the most congested. After passing the Girard Bridge, traffic will thin a bit.

Boathouse Row dates back to the founding of the Schuylkill Navy in 1858, and many of the houses are between 100 and 150 years old. The portion of river between the Girard Bridge and the Colombia Bridge is very popular for rowing, and depending on time of day, you may see graceful singles on calm waters or stunning eights finishing practice. Regattas take place on Sundays between the Colombia and Strawberry Mansion bridges.

After Strawberry Mansion, you'll pass Laurel Hill Cemetery, perched to the right of Kelly Drive. Laurel Hill celebrated its 175th anniversary in 2011. There are lots of familiar Philadelphia names here, including Rittenhouse, Widener, Elkins, and Strawbridge.

After crossing the Falls Bridge, you'll pick up a narrow path that runs alongside Martin Luther King Drive and heads back towards the Art Museum. Most of MLK Drive is closed to traffic on weekends during the summer, offering a wide stretch of road for runners and cyclists adorned with lush greenery. Hooray!

On this side of the river, you are treated to the best views of Boathouse Row, the waterworks, and the Art Museum. As you continue towards the museum, the path narrows still. After crossing the river again, you'll have to cross Benjamin Franklin Parkway to reach the entrance to Schuylkill Banks Park. If uncomfortable with the traffic, wait to cross at the stop light. You'll see the entrance to Schuylkill Banks Park just after the light – make a left if you wish to ride along the banks towards Locust Street (Ride 3), or a right if you want to head back towards Boathouse Row.

Now here is a totally awesome thing to add to your ride: The Fairmount Park Art Association recently released Museum Without Walls, an audio interpretation of the public art and sculpture along the Loop. The apps, maps, and audio downloads are available for 35 works of public art. If you plan to spend an afternoon on the river, they are definitely worth a listen!

Art Museum Departures

Ride Log

P1 Lloyd Hall
P2 Boathouse Row
P3 Philadelphia Zoo
P4 Columbia Bridge
P5 Laurel Hill Cemetery

B1 Fairmount Bicycles, 2015 Fairmount Ave
BR1 In-season bicycle rental stand

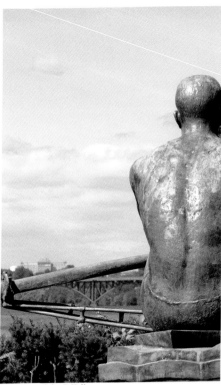

The Rower, John B Kelly.

0.0 Start at entrance to Schuylkill Banks Park, and head north. You'll immediately pedal down a short hill and under a small overhang.

0.2 Pass the waterworks to the left, and make a left to cross the little road. Pick up the path along the river, and make a right.

0.4 Make a left at Lloyd Hall to enter Boathouse Row.

0.7 The path splits after the Viking statue at the end of Boathouse Row. Follow the path street side (unless you want to tackle the river-side stairs!).

1.1 Pedal under Girard Bridge. This is a good spot to ring your bell.

1.6 You'll see the Playing Angels statue (best viewed at dusk) close to the river.

2.0 Pedal under the Columbia Bridge, past the Grandstand and John B. Kelly (The Rower) statue.

2.9 Pedal under Strawberry Mansion Bridge.

3.6 Pass Laurel Hill Cemetery to the right of Kelly Dr.

4.1 You'll see a series of bridges ahead. Make a left over the Falls Bridge, (the boxy, mint green number). Make another, immediate left after the bridge to pick up MLK Dr path.

4.2 Follow the path back towards the city. Bonus! MLK Dr is closed to traffic weekends in the summer.

5.2 Enjoy the path. Pass Belmont Stables to the right.

7.2 Pedal again under the Girard Bridge, and you'll notice that the path narrows considerably.

8.1 Follow the path alongside Ben Franklin Pkwy. This section feels like a sidewalk.

8.2 Cross Ben Franklin Pkwy at the stoplight to re-enter Schuylkill Banks Park.

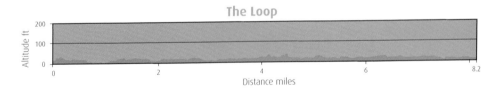

The Loop

Altitude ft

200
100
0

0   2   4   6   8.2

Distance miles

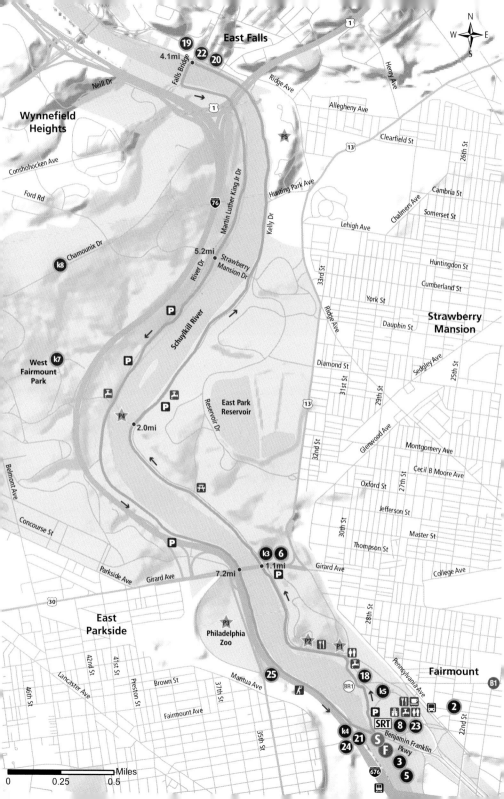

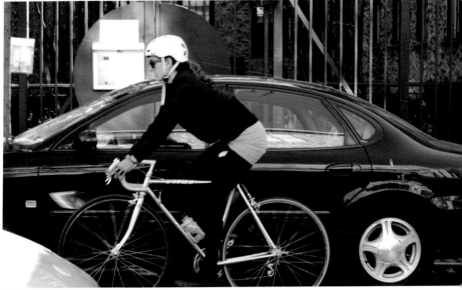

Biking alongside traffic in Manayunk.

At a Glance

Distance 5.4 miles   **Total Elevation** 93 feet

Terrain

The ride to Manayunk begins on the flat Schuylkill River Trail, and then moves across the softest of hills before reaching Main Street.

Traffic

After you turn off the SRT, there will be steady car traffic on Main Street. Cars are parked on both sides of the street here, so even though this is a heavily traveled bike corridor, make sure you watch out for the errant car door.

How to Get There

The starting point for this ride is just behind the Art Museum - Septa bus routes 7, 32, 38, 43 and 48 serve the museum area. If driving, you'll find ample parking behind the Art Museum and Boathouse Row.

Food and Drink

There are restaurants and cafés all along Main Street, many with outdoor seating. Le Bus and La Colombe are favorites.

Side Trip

Check out the Schuylkill Center for Environmental Education, just past the Ridge Avenue hill on Hagy's Mill Road. One of the first urban environmental education centers in the country, the Schuylkill center offers visitors 340 green acres, three miles of hiking trails and a variety of exhibits, courses, and speakers.

Links to ② ③ ⑤ ⑥ ⑧ ⑪ ⑫ ⑰ ⑲ ⑳ ㉑ ㉒ ㉓ ㉔ ㉕

Where to Bike Rating 🚲🚲🚲

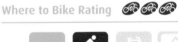

About...

Want to add a little something extra to the Loop? Head to Manayunk! This is a great ride for confident beginners who want to bike a little bit farther than they are accustomed to. Main Street acts as the prime connector between two portions of the SRT: Philadelphia and Valley Forge, so you'll be in good company, and there are a few bike shops in Manayunk that will help you change your first flat.

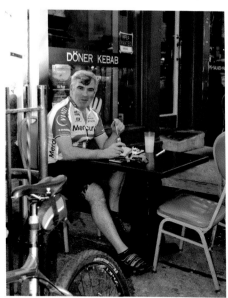
Eating on Main Street!

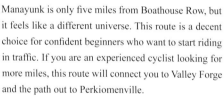

Manayunk is only five miles from Boathouse Row, but it feels like a different universe. This route is a decent choice for confident beginners who want to start riding in traffic. If you are an experienced cyclist looking for more miles, this route will connect you to Valley Forge and the path out to Perkiomenville.

You'll start along the river, heading away from the city. This part of the Schuylkill River Trail will become very familiar to you if you take up cycling in Philadelphia! You'll pass the Girard, Columbia and Strawberry Mansion bridges. But, rather than cross Falls Bridge to MLK Drive as in the Loop, you'll go straight across Calumet Street and head towards Ridge Avenue.

This section is more like a sidewalk than a path, and sometimes cyclists play chicken. It won't look like the rest of the SRT, but rest assured, you are heading in the correct direction.

Once you hit Ridge Avenue, you'll have to make a left turn to head towards Main Street (The Septa Wissahickon Transfer Center will be on the corner). You'll have two options here – take the hard left, which will put you on the path towards Main Street, Manayunk (you will see an enormous sign beckoning you towards Manayunk). There are a couple of bus lanes that you

can abuse to make your way over to Main Street. If you make a mistake and take the soft left, you will find yourself heading up the very long, and very steep Ridge Avenue Hill, and probably cursing me under your breath.

You will pass a movie theater to your right and then a few revitalized warehouses. The shops, restaurants and cafés that line Main Street are just ahead. The streets get more congested along this strip and there are also quite a few stoplights. If you haven't cycled in traffic before, take it slow. If you feel like riding farther, you'll find an entrance to the gravel towpath just off Lock Street. Or just lock up your bikes and walk around town.

Consider waking up early on a Saturday and riding out here for brunch – it's a great way to spend the morning and the traffic will be lighter!

Ride Log

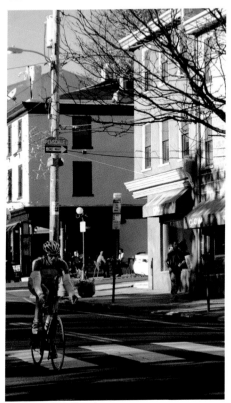

Pedaling on Main Street!

P1 Playing Angels Statue
P2 Regatta Grandstand
P3 Laurel Hill Cemetery

B1 Cadence Performance Cycling,
4323 Main Street
B2 Human Zoom, 4159 Main Street
B3 Fairmount Bicycles, 2015 Fairmount Ave

Hop on your bike anywhere on the Schuylkill River Trail near Lloyd Hall. The ride log begins at Boathouse Row.

0.0 Start out on the Schuylkill River Trail heading towards the Viking Statue at the end of Boathouse Row. You'll be riding northwest. Follow the path as you would if you were to do the Loop (Ride 17).

0.6 Pass under the Girard Bridge, and continue to follow the path.

1.5 Pedal under the Columbia Bridge, past the grandstand and John B. Kelly (The Rower) statue.

2.5 Pass under the Strawberry Mansion Bridge.

3.6 The boxy, mint colored Falls Bridge will be to your left. Cross Calumet St and continue on the narrow path ahead.

4.1 Pass under two highway overhangs and follow the curve to the right; the path will feel like a sidewalk.

4.4 Make a left on Ridge Ave and then bear left. You will be heading towards Main St in Manayunk (FYI the entrance to Forbidden Dr – Ride 12 is just across Ridge Ave). There is a huge sign over the street directing you towards Manayunk. This is a heavily traveled bicycle route, and there are some decent shoulders here, but it can be awkward to bear left while moving to the right side of the street.

4.8 Cruise along Main St Manayunk. There will be steady car traffic, but also plenty of cyclists.

5.2 You are now in the heart Manayunk. Welcome!

5.4 The entrance to the Tow Path (Ride 11) is by the river, just off Lock St. Le Bus, a café and bakery is just past Rector St. La Colombe, aka the city's best coffee roaster, is just after Grape St. Swap to the log for Ride 19 if you'd like to venture further on towards Valley Forge.

The Art Museum to Manayunk

Altitude ft

Distance miles

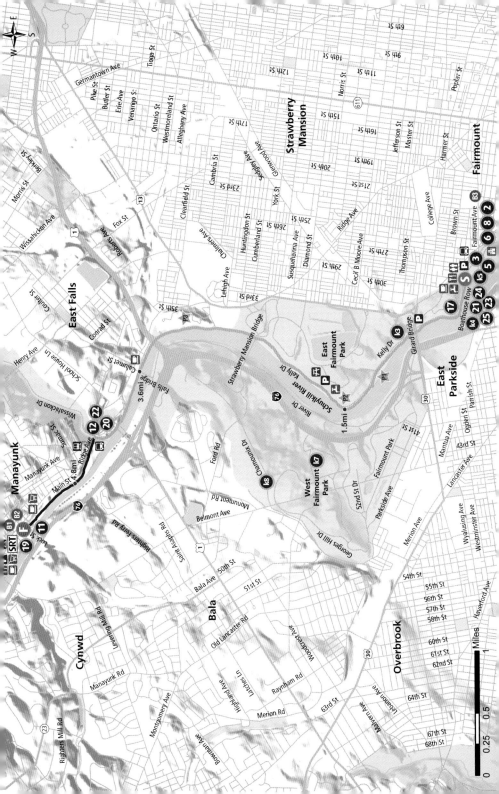

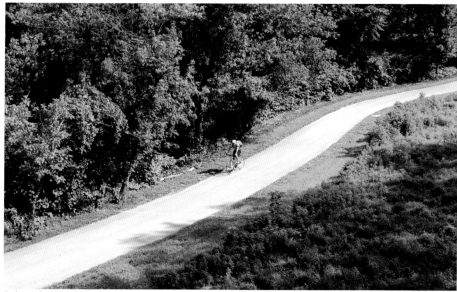

Riding solo along the SRT.

At a Glance

Distance 20.6 miles   **Total Elevation** 199 feet

Terrain

For most of the trip, you'll ride on the Schuylkill River Trail, an off-road, paved path. However some trail connections are not yet complete and you will be on-road for a bit through Manayunk.

Traffic

This is a pretty popular ride – though there will be a decent amount of car traffic through Manayunk, plenty of cyclists will join you between Ridge Avenue and Umbria Street. Once on the path, there will be a steady flow of bicycles.

How to Get There

Septa bus routes 7, 32, 38, 43 and 48 serve the museum area. If driving, you'll find ample parking behind the Art Museum and Boathouse Row. The Manayunk/Norristown Regional Rail line runs parallel to the Valley Forge section of the Schuylkill River Trail in the event of poop-out.

Food and Drink

You'll pass tons of places to stop for a bite or a cup of coffee on Main Street in Manayunk, including Le Bus and La Colombe. The Spring Mill Café is just off the path on Barren Hill Road in Conshohocken. But be sure to pack extra water for the rest of the trail to Valley Forge!

Side Trip

The Valley Forge National Historical Park, with its stunning landscape, monuments and shaded paths, is an excellent place to picnic or spend the afternoon. The entrance is just across Route 23 (see Ride 26 for details).

Links to ② ③ ⑤ ⑥ ⑧ ⑪ ⑫ ⑰ ⑱ ⑳ ㉑ ㉒ ㉓ ㉔ ㉕ ㉖ ㉗ ㉘ ㉙

Where to Bike Rating

About...

This tried and true ride comes highly recommended by droves of city cyclists. It is pretty straight forward, offering a couple of good hills in Manayunk and a flat and fast path through to Valley Forge. You also have the option of picking up the towpath in Manayunk if not comfortable on the busy Main Street. A word of caution – I've gotten more flats on this route than any others in the city. Bring some extra tubes!

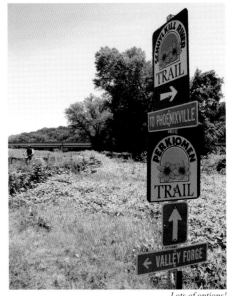

Lots of options!

Art Museum Departures

The great thing about this ride is that you can go for as long as you wish, and when sufficiently cycled out, you can return along the same route or hop on the Manayunk/Norristown line to hitch home. If making a realxed day out of it, then you should lock up your bikes and stroll through the 'Yunk; there are lots of lovely shops and cafes to visit in this part of town. If clad in Spandex, you will enjoy the ability to extend this ride quite a bit farther by utilizing the trail network just beyond Valley Forge National Historical Park.

You'll start off as with most other Art Museum Departures, heading north along the Loop. After Falls Bridge, you'll continue along the river until Ridge Avenue, where you'll make a sharp left to head into Manayunk. There are two options for you: the on-road Main Street/Umbria route, and the towpath (Ride 11). Umbria has traffic and a nice hill. The towpath is packed gravel and can sometimes be muddy.

At about mile eight, you'll pick up The Schuylkill River Trail to Valley Forge. Try to stay on the section that leads to the right and pass on the left here – this path can be very busy on the weekends, and it isn't terribly wide. Some sections are green and shaded, others are sunny and hot in the warmer months. Bring extra

water! Extra tubes!

The path will take you along the rail line through Miquon, Spring Mill, Conshohocken, and Norristown. At about mile 15, you'll pass the Norristown Transportation Center – the last on the line. Many times I've been caught in the weather and happily hopped on the train to head home.

Once in Valley Forge, you have quite a few options to extend the ride. For starters, there is a good network of paved trails in the Valley Forge National Historical Park (Ride 26). There is also the Audubon Loop (Ride 28), offering a challenging nine percent grade hill. If you want to be bold, take the Perkiomen Trail (Ride 27) all the way out to Perkiomenville. Just remember to turn around!

Ride Log

0.0 Start by the viking statue at the end of Boathouse Row, and head northwest along the river.

0.4 Pass under Girard Bridge, and continue to follow the path.

3.4 The Falls Bridge will be to your left. Cross Calumet St and continue on the narrow path ahead.

3.9 Pass under two highway overhangs and follow the curve to the right; the path will feel like a sidewalk.

4.2 Make a left on Ridge Ave and then bear left to head towards Main St Manayunk.

4.3 Cruise along Main St. Le Bus, a café and bakery is just past Rector St. La Colombe, aka the city's best coffee roaster, is just after Grape St.

5.8 Right on Leverington St (a little climb here) just after Green Ln.

5.9 Quick left on Umbria St. At Wilde St you've gone too far!

6.3 Pickup the Umbria St bike lanes, with a hill ahead

7.4 Follow Umbria's curve to the right, then take the Shawmont Ave switchback (nice downhill!).

7.6 Make a right on Nixon St.

7.9 Pop up the Port Royal Ave hill and make a left to enter the Valley Forge section of the Schuylkill River Trail.

8.9 Pass the Miquon train station.

10.5 Pass the Spring Mill station.

11.7 Pass the Conshohocken station.

14.6 Follow the loopdiloop around.

15.6 Pass the Norristown Transportation Center – last stop on the Norristown/Manayunk line.

16.4 Cross Haws Ave.

18.0 Cross S Schuylkill Ave.

18.3 Cross Port Indian Rd.

 P1 Valley Forge National Historical Park
1400 North Outerline Drive, King of Prussia

 B1 Cadence Cycling, 3423 Main St, Philadelphia
B2 The Bike Stop, 1987 W Main St, Eagleville

20.5 Cross W County Line Rd, and enter Valley Forge National Historical Park. Finally some shade!

20.6 Reach the Betzwood picnic area. To reach Ride 27 or 28, keep on heading straight through the park until you pop out at the Pawlings Rd intersection. To reach Ride 26, which begins at the Valley Forge National Historical Park visitor center, you'll have to cross the Schuylkill River by taking the Rt 422 bridge. Make a left when you reach Rt 23 and head up the hill to reach the visitor center. Or, turn yourself around and head back to Philly!

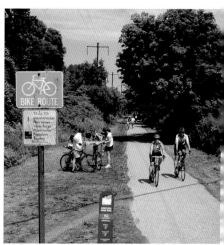

Entrance to the Valley Forge Trail.

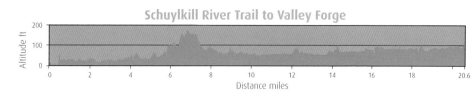

Schuylkill River Trail to Valley Forge

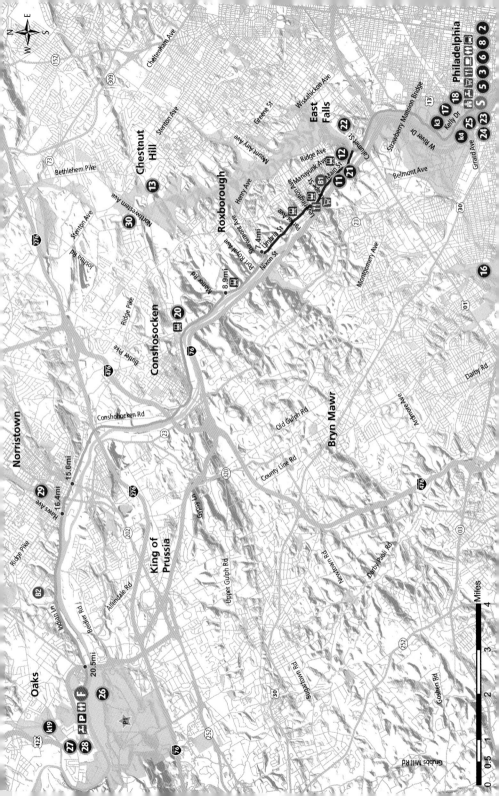

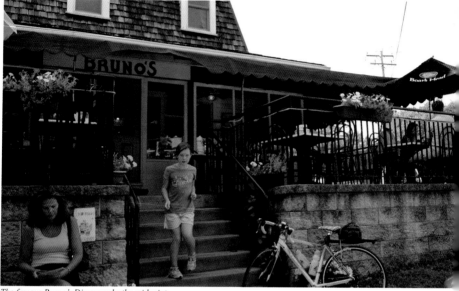

The famous Bruno's Diner marks the midpoint.

At a Glance

Distance 27.3 miles   **Total Elevation** 418 feet

Terrain

This ride takes you on road through Chestnut Hill, which, as the name implies, has one very large hill. You'll encounter some climbing along the way and a few luxurious downhills.

Traffic

Most of the roads are quiet, though a couple (including Ridge and Henry avenues), will have steady traffic. Bike lanes pop up here and there, as does a few miles of the Schuylkill River Trail.

How to Get There

The log begins at Lloyd Hall on Kelly Drive. Septa bus routes 7, 32, 38, 43 and 48 serve the museum area. If driving, you'll find ample parking behind the Art Museum and Boathouse Row.

Food and Drink

Bruno's, a neighborhood diner with great food, marks the halfway point of this loop. There is a small ice cream shop next door as well.

Side Trip

Morris Arboretum of course! Talk about a place to lose yourself for an afternoon – the gorgeous historic gardens span 92 acres and contain sculptures, lovely walkways and streams, in addition to over 13,000 labeled plants, flowers and stately trees.

Links to ② ③ ⑤ ⑥ ⑧ ⑪ ⑫ ⑬ ⑰ ⑱ ⑲ ㉑ ㉒ ㉓ ㉔ ㉕ ㉚

Where to Bike Rating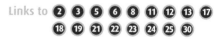

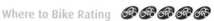

About...

The ride from Center City to Bruno's in Chestnut Hill is a longstanding tradition for the Bicycle Club of Philadelphia. Many versions exist, but from what I understand, this one is the classic (thanks to the folks at BCP for finding the best roads!). You'll cover a lot of ground on an array of streets – some are busy urban arterials, while others seem like slow country roads – before finishing up with a few miles on the SRT and a quick jaunt through Manayunk.

This is a great ride if you are ready for something more advanced but would still like the comfort of knowing that there are poop out options along the way. The full ride is a solid 27 miles, but for you, the non-committal rider, it can be shortened to 11 miles by catching the Chestnut Hill West line at Highland Avenue back to Center City, or to 16 miles by taking the Manayunk/Norristown line at Spring Mill. So go for it!

The majority of this ride is on quieter roads, though a few will have steady traffic. Most have a wide shoulder. There are a handful of bridges to cross and circles to navigate, but if you take your time, relax, and follow the flow of traffic, you shouldn't encounter any trouble.

The first portion of this ride takes you from Boathouse Row to Chestnut Hill, a quiet neighborhood with beautiful old houses and big trees in the northwestern section of the city. There are a few good climbs and busy streets, most notably Ridge Avenue, Henry Avenue, and Germantown Avenue, but you will not be on these roads for long.

Bruno's is on the corner of Northwestern and Germantown avenues. If you wish to make a day of the trip and visit Morris Arboretum, simply make a right on Northwestern. The entrance to the arboretum is just

down the hill.

There are two options for your return – Forbidden Drive (Ride 12) or the long way through Manayunk. The second portion of your ride, should you choose the long way, all leads up to the very long, rolling Barren Hill Road. This is by far the loveliest road on the ride. After a few turns, you'll pick up The Schuylkill River Trail and ride towards the city.

The third portion of this head brings you up Umbria Street and down Main Street in Manayunk. Main Street will have steady traffic, but drivers are generally accustomed to seeing cyclists (Umbria is the main connection between the Kelly Drive portion of the SRT and the Valley Forge portion). After your ride through Manayunk, you'll pick up the loop along Kelly Drive and bike back to the boathouses.

And don't forget…The Bicycle Club of Philadelphia is always looking for new members! Check out their ride calendar online at www.bikeclubphilly.org.

Ride Log

0.0 Start at Lloyd Hall on Boathouse Row, and head away from the city.

0.6 Pass under Girard Bridge, and continue to follow the path.

3.6 The Falls Bridge will be to your left. Cross Calumet St and continue on the narrow path ahead.

4.4 Make a right on Ridge Ave. This intersection can be confusing on your first approach.

5.2 Left on Midvale.

5.6 Left on Warden Dr, the Schuylkill Free Library is on the corner.

5.9 Left on Vaux St.

6.0 Right on School House Ln.

6.1 Left on Henry Ave at the stoplight. Be careful here - this is the busiest street of the route.

6.5 Cross the Henry Ave Bridge.

7.1 Right on Walnut St to pick up a small bike lane. Follow bike lanes over the bridge.

7.7 Bike around the circle and make a left on Park Line Dr.

Ride Log

8.0 Right on Hortter St. Cross Wissahickon Ave.

8.3 Left on Wayne and pick up the bike lanes.

8.8 Right onto Sedgwick St.

8.9 Left on Sherman St, around the park. Sherman becomes Mt Pleasant Rd.

9.3 Make a left on McCallum St and follow it over the bridge (there are sidewalks on the bridge if you are uncomfortable with the traffic).

10.0 After the bridge, you'll make a right on Mermaid Ln.

10.05 Take the first left on Cherokee St.

10.3 Pass Springside School and bear right. Cherokee becomes Hartwell Ln.

10.9 Left on St Martins Ln.

11.3 Left on Seminole St. If pooped out, hop on the Chestnut Hill West line at Highland Ave back to the city.

11.5 Right on Chestnut Hill Ave.

11.7 Left on Crefeld Ave. Bear right at the stop, and Crefeld Ave becomes Normal Ln. Go up the hill!

12.0 Left on Germantown Ave, one of the busier streets on this route. Enjoy the downhill!

13.1 Bruno's! The favorite diner is on the corner of Northwestern and Germantown avenues.

Return: you can either take Forbidden Dr home (Ride 12), or enjoy the following route home through Manayunk.

13.2 Stay on Northwestern. The entrance to Forbidden Dr is on your left. If going through Manayunk home, then:

13.3 Right on Andorra Rd.

14.3 Make a sharp right on Park Rd, and a quick left on

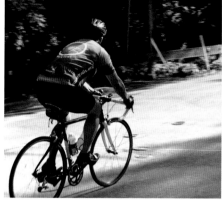

Andorra Road.

Church Rd (becomes Hart Ln).

14.8 Right on Barren Hill Rd – a beautiful road but small shoulder. Take this all the way to the bottom!

16.1 Pass Spring Mill Café, follow curve to the right. Make a left at the light on Hector St.

16.4 Left on North Ln. Follow signs for the bike path. If pooped out, hop on the Spring Mill R6 home.

16.5 Make a left to pick up the Schuylkill River Trail.

19.1 Exit path and bike down the short hill on Nixon St.

19.4 Right on Shawmont, up and around the switchback to reach the Umbria St bike lanes.

21.1 Make a right at the T, and follow Umbria under the bridge and to the left. Umbria becomes Main St.

22.6 Merge with Ridge Ave, stay to the right.

22.9 Right to pick up the Schuylkill River Trail. Stay on the trail until you reach Boathouse Row.

27.3 Finish!

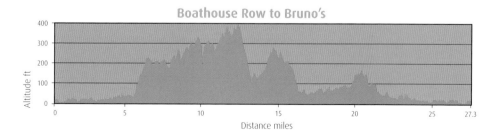

Boathouse Row to Bruno's

Altitude ft

Distance miles

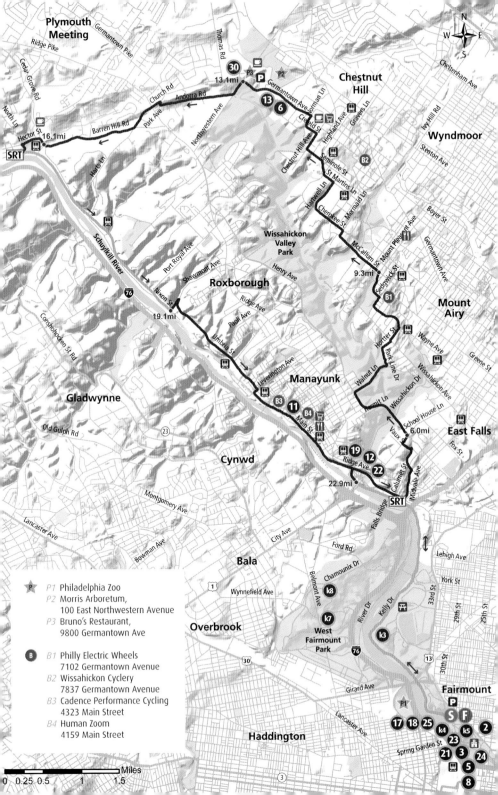

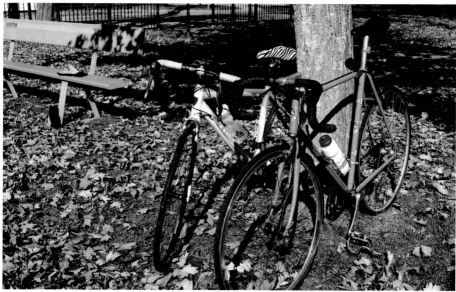

Fall in Bryn Mawr.

At a Glance

Distance 24.4 miles   **Total Elevation** 425 feet

Terrain

This ride is mostly on-road, with a few paved paths sprinkled in between. It's super hilly and makes for a great workout.

Traffic

The roads you'll take are very amenable to bicycle travel, including the roads in Fairmount Park and those out farther on the Mainline. There will be a bit more car traffic along Route 23 and through Manayunk.

How to Get There

The starting point for this ride is just behind the Art Museum – Septa bus routes 7, 32, 38, 43 and 48 serve the museum area. If driving, you'll find ample parking behind the Art Museum and Boathouse Row.

Food and Drink

You'll ride by a convenience store every few miles,

and there are lots of lunch options in Manayunk. Of course, we waited until Boathouse Row for a fresh soft pretzel from Chief (see Ride 17). A new spot – Cosmic Foods – just opened at Lloyd Hall.

Side Trip

Take some time to explore West Fairmount Park – you'll be very close to the Please Touch Museum, the Whispering Bench, the Horticulture Center, the Japanese House and Garden, and the gorgeous lookout from the Belmont Mansion.

Links to ② ③ ⑤ ⑥ ⑧ ⑪ ⑫ ⑰ ⑱ ⑲ ⑳ ㉒ ㉓ ㉔ ㉕

Where to Bike Rating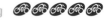

About...

Take this ride! The mega-hilly loop runs from West Fairmount Park out to Bala Cynwyd, Bryn Mawr, and Gladwyne. You'll hit the biggest ups and downs in the book, then follow the Schuylkill for a bit before crossing the river and riding through Manayunk on your way back to the city. This ride comes to you care of my dear friend Joel Flood, a longtime Philadelphia cyclist and lover of bringing vintage bicycles up insane inclines.

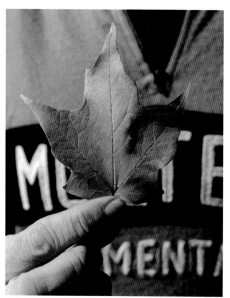

Joel's sweater matches the foliage.

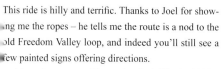

This ride is hilly and terrific. Thanks to Joel for showing me the ropes – he tells me the route is a nod to the old Freedom Valley loop, and indeed you'll still see a few painted signs offering directions.

Along the way, you'll see what feels like the hidden side of everything. It almost seems like a secret. You'll start out along Martin Luther King Drive and wind your way through West Fairmount Park. With just a few turns, you'll find yourself riding through the shady residential roads of Bala Cynwyd and Bryn Mawr.

Some streets will seem to go on for days, among them are Bryn Mawr Avenue, Old Gulf Road, and Youngsford Road. There will be a handful of forks along the way, so unless you are positive that it is time to turn, be sure to follow the signs and stick to the riding log on these roads.

The highlight of this loop comes right around mile 12: a long downhill that brings you all the way from the 'burbs to the edge of the Schuylkill. You'll then be treated to about a mile and a half of flat pedaling alongside the river, a stretch that offers a gorgeous quiet view of the water. Then you have to snap to – and fast – you're about to go up the most challenging hill in this guidebook: Hollow Road.

Hollow Road is a beast. You'll head uphill for close to a mile, make a left on Route 23, and then crawl up another half mile incline. I would not attempt this hill if you are even mildly hungover, as I was, on the morning I went up Hollow Road with Joel. Fair warning!

After Hollow Road, the rest of the loop is pretty much downhill. You'll cross the Schuylkill and find yourself surprised by just how close you've been this whole time to Manayunk (for more info about this neighborhood, check out rides 11 and 18). You'll ride on through Main Street and then pick up the Schuylkill River Trail off Ridge Avenue. The final leg is a common one in this book – hoofing it back to the Boathouse Row via Kelly Drive. You'll be ready for a massive lunch!

Ride Log

P1 Philadelphia Zoo
P2 Chamounix Mansion
P3 The big hill on Hollow Road

B1 Fairmount Bicycles
2015 Fairmount Ave, Philadelphia PA 19130
B2 Cadence Performance Cycling
4323 Main Street, Philadelphia PA 19127
B3 Human Zoom
4159 Main Street, Philadelphia
B4 Main Line Cycles
717 Montgomery Ave, Narberth

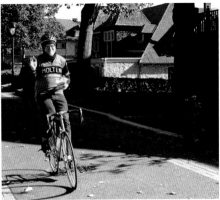

Thanks for a great ride, Joles!

0.0 Start out behind the Art Museum where the Schuylkill River Trail meets Schuylkill Banks. Hop on MLK Dr and head up river.

3.1 Left on Greenland Dr, and follow the switchback.

3.6 Left on Chamounix Dr.

4.5 Bear right on Belmont Mansion Dr and cross Belmont Ave.

4.7 Left on Parkside Ave.

5.0 Right on Wynnefield Ave.

5.3 Right on Bryn Mawr Ave.

6.4 Cross Montgomery Ave, continue on Bryn Mawr Ave.

7.4 Follow the curve left in Bryn Mawr Ave.

8.5 Right on Old Gulf Rd. Continue to follow Old Gulf for a ways.

10.0 Bear right on Merion Square Rd.

10.8 Right on Youngsford Rd. There will be a few forks, but just keep on Youngsford.

11.6 Right on Waverly Rd.

12.11 Bear left to continue on Waverly. You are about to hit one of the best downhills in the book – all the way down to the river.

12.8 Right on River Rd to follow the Schuylkill.

14.3 Right on Hollow Rd – one of the hardest uphills around.

15.4 Left on Rt 23. And, there's a little bit more hill ahead.

17.0 Left on Rock Hill Rd.

17.6 Left on Belmont Ave.

17.7 Bear Left at the fork to follow Old Belmont Ave.

17.9 Cross the Schuylkill.

18.0 Right on Main St Manayunk. Follow Main St until it becomes Ridge Ave.

19.5 Make a right just past the Septa transfer station to pick up the Schuylkill River Trail.

20.0 Pass Falls Bridge and ride on home.

23.8 Hang a right at the end of Boathouse Row to head towards the Waterworks.

24.4 Ride under the Spring Garden Bridge and bam! You are back to where you started.

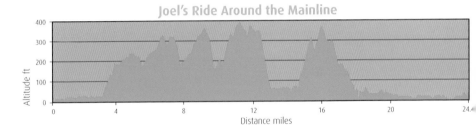

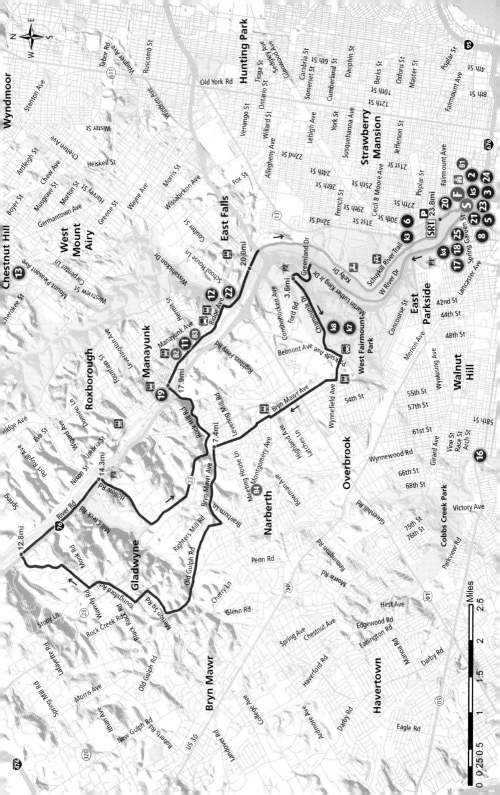

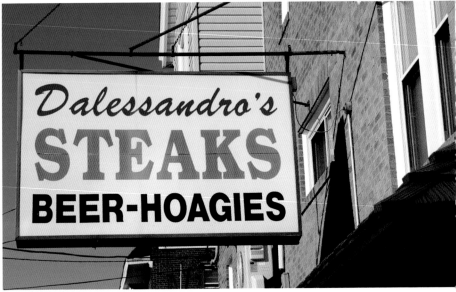

So GOOD!

At a Glance

Distance 7.2 miles   **Total Elevation** 240 feet

Terrain

This one-way ticket to Dalessandro's takes advantage of the Schuylkill River Trail before moving on-road through East Falls.

Traffic

The SRT will have heavy bike/ped traffic as usual. Ridge and Henry avenues will have steady traffic, but the other streets are fairly quiet.

How to Get There

The log begins at Lloyd Hall on Kelly Drive. Septa bus routes 7, 32, 38, 43 and 48 serve the museum area. If driving, you'll find ample parking behind the Art Museum and Boathouse Row.

Food and Drink

Duh. The whole point of this trip is to use human powered transport to get yourself one of the best steaks in

the city: Dalessandro's.

Side Trip

After eating one of these incredible sandwiches, you might feel the urge to have a bit more physical activity. You could easily spend the afternoon riding down Forbidden Drive (Ride 12) or hiking in the surrounding woods there.

Links to ② ③ ⑤ ⑥ ⑧ ⑫ ⑰ ⑱ ⑲ ⑳
㉑ ㉓ ㉔ ㉕

Where to Bike Rating

About...

The trip to Dalessandro's, which is in the Roxborough section of Philadelphia, is seven miles from Boathouse Row. You'll take the SRT and then have a bit of on-road pedaling as you get closer to lunch. This is the second of WTB Philly's Cheesesteak Rides; you can ride to the first (John's Roast Pork) by connecting this log to rides 3, 1 and 9. Belly. Ache!

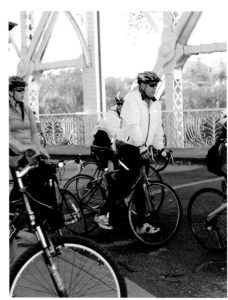

Busy bike intersection at Falls Bridge.

Try this ride for a simple 14 mile loop. You'll get yourself a bit out of the city and enjoy an amazing cheesesteak to boot.

As with many of the other Kelly Drive departures, this one begins near Boathouse Row. You'll pedal up river for the first 4.5 miles, passing the Girard, Columbia, Strawberry Mansion, and Falls bridges. As usual, this stretch of the river will be busy in the warmer months, and downright crowded on weekends. Be sure to take your time and call out when passing.

Once on Ridge Avenue, you'll make a right to head towards East Falls. This corner has a lot of traffic, and I can't recall a time when there wasn't construction, so use a bit of caution here. You'll ride along Ridge for about three-quarters of a mile before turning up Midvale.

The next set of streets (Midvale, Warden, Vaux, and School House) are much quieter. There is a steady incline here for about a mile, but you'll be able to catch your breath by School House.

Henry Avenue is coming up next, and it is busy. You'll make a left by Philadelphia University – make sure to get in the turn lane. If you don't mind riding in traffic, then Henry won't be a problem, but if you're new to this sort of thing you might be uncomfortable the first few times. You'll ride over the Henry Avenue Bridge as well, which again depending on your cycling confidence, you will enjoy or dislike very, very much.

Once over the bridge, look for Walnut Lane. You should be smelling cheesesteaks heavy in the air by now – just ahead on the corner of Henry Avenue and Wendover you'll see Chubby's Steaks on the left and Dalessandro's on the right. Park your bike and eat up.

Feel like a cheesesteak challenge? You can connect this ride Schuylkill Banks Park (Ride 3), Center City Bike Lane Heaven (Ride 1) and Cheesesteak Ride #1 (Ride 9) to pedal all the way from Dalessandro's in Roxborough to Tony Luke's in South Philadelphia.

Ride Log

0.0 Start at Lloyd Hall on Boathouse Row, and head upriver.

0.6 Pass under Girard Bridge. Continue to follow the path.

1.6 Follow the bend in the river around Columbia Bridge. Pass the regatta grandstand.

3.6 The Falls Bridge will be to your left. Cross Calumet St and continue on the narrow path ahead.

4.1 Pass under two highway overhangs and follow the path. It will feel like a sidewalk.

4.4 Make a right on Ridge Ave. This intersection can be confusing on your first approach. Follow the signs for Ridge and take advantage of the stoplights.

5.2 Make a left on Midvale, (Midvale is just after Eveline St, just before Indian Queen Ln).

5.6 Left on Warden Dr, the Schuylkill Free Library is on the corner. There's a nice wide shoulder on Warden.

5.9 Left on Vaux St.

6.0 Right on School House Ln.

6.1 Left on Henry Ave at the stoplight. You'll be close to Philadelphia University. Henry Avenue is the busiest street of the route, so be sure to use caution.

6.5 Cross the Henry Ave Bridge. Caution here too.

7.1 The smell of Cheesesteaks begins to hang low in the air. Cross Walnut Ln.

7.2 Arrive at Dalessandro's, on the corner of Henry Ave and Wendover St.

P1 Philadelphia Zoo
P2 Regatta Grandstand
P3 Philadelphia University
P4 Henry Avenue Bridge

B *B1* Fairmount Bicycles, 2015 Fairmount Ave
B2 Cadence Performance Cycling, 4323 Main Street
B3 Human Zoom, 4159 Main Street
BR *BR1* In-season bicycle rental stand

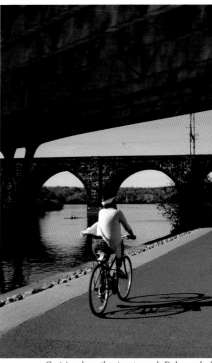

Cruising down the river towards Dalessandro's

Cheesesteak Ride #2: Dalessandro's

Altitude ft / Distance miles

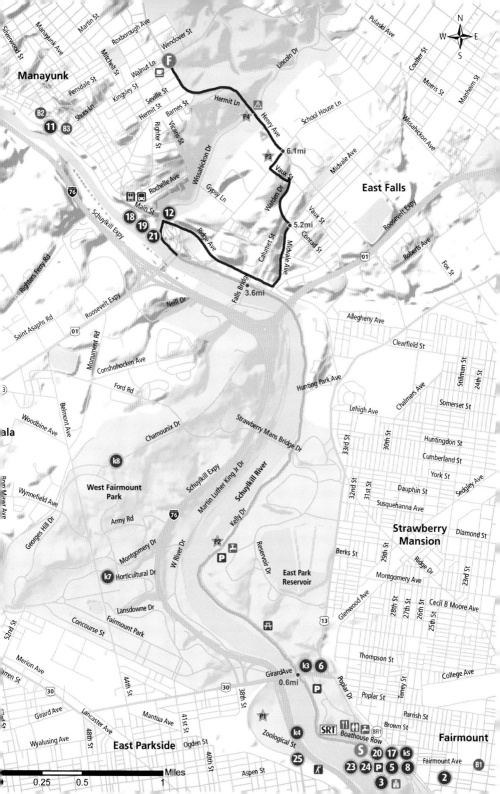

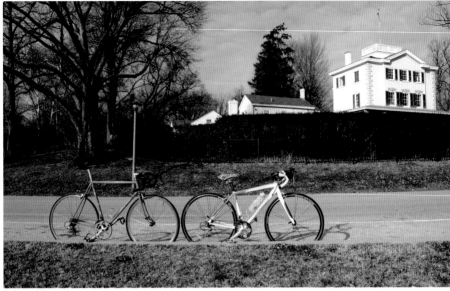

Belmont Mansion.

At a Glance

Park Ride

Distance 12.5 miles   **Total Elevation** 281 feet

Terrain

A mix of on-road cycling and bike paths through West Fairmount Park, this loop has a couple of spiky hills and one long, luxurious downhill at mile six.

Traffic

The bike paths around West Fairmount Park are far less utilized than the Schuylkill River Trail, which is on the east side of the river. Car traffic is generally low during the on road portions, but there are a few hairy intersections to watch (specifically Belmont Mansion Drive and Montgomery Avenue).

How to Get There

The ride starts at the corner of 22nd and Spring Garden. Buses 7, 43, and 48 will get you close to 22nd and Spring Garden, which is near the Art Museum. There is also ample street parking in the Fairmount neighborhood.

Food and Drink

Grab a snack at the shop on 22nd and Spring Garden because you won't have many opportunities for a bit until you reach The Chief at Boathouse Row!

Side Trip

Check out all the mansions along the way! You can also take a tour of the Underground Railroad Museum at Belmont Mansion. Admission is $7.

Links to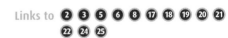

Where to Bike Rating

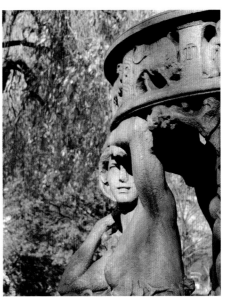

About...

Never ventured into West Fairmount Park? Give this 12 mile loop a go! It provides an excellent introduction to the area, brings you over the Falls Bridge, and then takes you back to Boathouse Row along the Schuylkill River Trail. You'll pass four beautiful historic mansions nestled in the park, including Cedar Grove, Sweetbriar, Belmont, and Chamounix. Belmont Mansion sits on the Belmont Plateau, an awesome stop that offers one of the best views of the Philadelphia skyline.

Lovely grounds by the Horticulture Center.

Start out on 22nd and Spring Garden and head towards the Art Museum. You'll ride in front of the museum steps on Ben Franklin Parkway on your way to Martin Luther King Drive, which is on the west side of the river (you'll see a street sign for "Schuylkill Trail Connector"). This ride shares its starting point with Ride 2 (Spring Garden to The Italian Market) – combine the two for a decent 20 mile loop that runs from Falls Bridge to The Italian Market. Not bad!

After you pick up MLK Drive, you'll head north along the river and, after about a mile, you'll make a left at Sweet Briar to head into the park – this will be your first uphill. You'll pick up the bike lanes as you pass Cedar Grove and Sweetbriar mansions. Both offer daily tours. Sweetbriar was built by Samuel Breck in the mid 19th century, and Cedar Grove was built in 1748 by Elizabeth Coates Pascall. The home was moved one brick at a time from its original location in Frankford to its current perch in the early part of the 20th century!

As you continue, you'll pass the back of the Please Touch Museum, and then the Shofuso Japanese House and Garden and the Horticulture Center. Soon you'll come to the intersection of Belmont Drive and Mont-gomery Avenue – depending on the time of day, it may take a few minutes to find a space in traffic long enough to cross the street. Take your time here at this intersection.

Once safely across, you'll hit another hill on your way up to the Belmont Plateau. This particular hill can be miserable on a hot afternoon with a single speed, but once you get there, the view is so amazing. Take a look at that beautiful city! The Belmont Mansion, which stoically sits behind you, was built in the 1700s. According to Fairmount Park Commission, Franklin, Jefferson, Washington, and Madison all hung out up here.

The last mansion you'll visit is the Chamounix Mansion, a country retreat built in 1802 by George Plumstead. It is currently a guesthouse – you can spend the night in Fairmount Park for less than $20 per person.

After Chamounix, you'll take the long downhill on Ford Road back towards the river. Cross either at Strawberry Mansion or Falls Bridge (the ride log takes you over Falls) to ride home along the Schuylkill River Trail on the east side of the river.

Ride Log

0.0 Start off at 22nd and Spring Garden. Make a left on Spring Garden and circle in front of the Art Museum to pick up Ben Franklin Pkwy. Cross the river on the Ben Franklin Pkwy and head towards MLK Dr. Right on MLK Dr to bike along the west side of the river.

1.8 Left on Sweet Briar (at the light).

1.9 Right onto bike path at Landsdown Dr.

2.2 Follow the curve in the bike path.

2.4 Make a right on Sweetbriar Dr to visit the Sweetbriar Mansion. Afterwards, continue along the bike path.

2.7 Pass the Cedar Grove Mansion.

3.0 Follow signs for the Please Touch Museum.

3.2 Pass the Shofuso Japanese House and Garden.

3.3 Right on Horticultural Dr and wrap around the Horticulture Center.

3.8 Right on Belmont Mansion Dr. Caution as you cross Montgomery, and up the hill you go!

4.3 Pass the Belmont Mansion atop the Belmont Plateau – awesome view!

4.5 Right on Chamounix Dr.

5.7 Pass the Chamounix Equestrian Center.

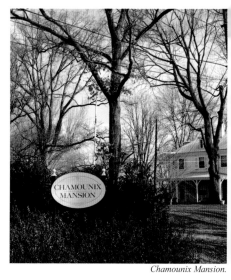
Chamounix Mansion.

5.8 Chamounix Mansion! Double Back along Chamounix Dr.

6.5 Left on Ford Rd. There is a fantastic downhill here.

7.0 Left on MLK Jr Dr. (If you want to cut the trip short, hop over the Strawberry Mansion Bridge and pick up the SRT towards Boathouse Row).

8.0 Make a right at Falls Bridge to cross the river.

8.1 Make another right after the bridge to pick up the SRT. Bike along the river for a final stretch until you reach Boathouse Row.

12.1 Pick up Pennsylvania Ave near the Art Museum by making a left and then a quick right.

12.4 Merge onto Spring Garden.

12.5 Back at 22nd and Spring Garden.

P P1 Sweetbriar Mansion
   P2 Cedar Grove Mansion
   P3 Please Touch Museum
   P4 Horticulture Center
   P5 Shofuso Japanese House & Garden
   P6 Belmont Mansion
   P7 Chamounix Mansion
   P8 Regatta Grandstand

B B1 Fairmount Bicycles, 2015 Fairmount Ave

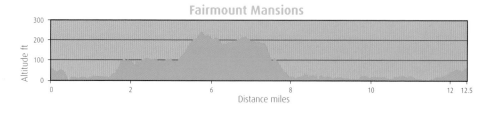

Fairmount Mansions

(chart: Altitude ft vs Distance miles)

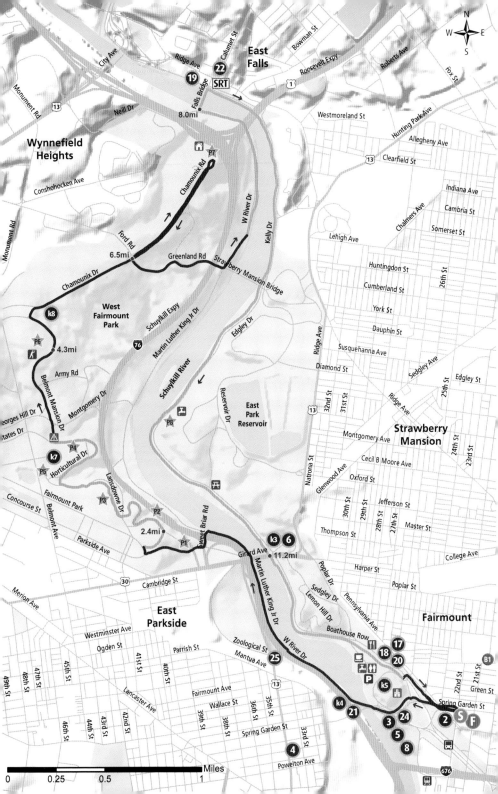

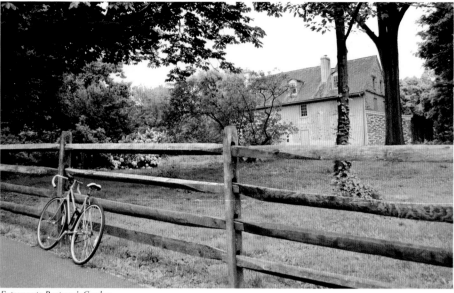

Entrance to Bartram's Garden.

At a Glance

Distance 7.8 miles   **Total Elevation** 105 feet

Terrain

Mostly flat with a few short hills. Watch out for the unrelenting maze of trolley tracks in West Philly!

Traffic

This ride is a hodgepodge of bike paths, bike lanes, and side streets. Some of the streets are very urban, and though both trolleys and cars will be rolling alongside of you, there should be room for you to ride on the right side.

How to Get There

You'll find a ramp to the Spring Garden bike lanes across the street from the entrance to Schuylkill Banks Park on the Ben Franklin Parkway. There is parking behind the Art Museum as well, if driving. Septa bus routes 7, 32, 38, 43 and 48 serve the museum area.

Food and Drink

You'll find a lot of great food trucks around the Penn campus. My favorite is the Magic Carpet Truck, parked at 34th and Walnut – just look out for the one with the longest line! There are also some good spots on Sansom Row and all along Spruce Street.

Side Trip

The Penn Museum of Archaeology and Anthropology is located at 33rd and South, just after Spruce Street. The collection has grown with each of the 400 expeditions that the museum has conducted since 1887, the year that the museum was founded.

Links to ❷ ❸ ❽ ❹ ❺ ❻ ⑰ ⑱ ⑲ ⑳ ㉑ ㉒ ㉓ ㉕

Where to Bike Rating 🚲🚲🚲🚲🚲

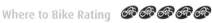

About...

The ride from the Art Museum to Bartram's Garden in West Philadelphia is definitely for the more adventurous cyclist. You'll enjoy such Philadelphia classics as trolley tracks and double parked cars, especially on Woodland Avenue. But wow, is the lovely Bartram's Garden ever worth it! This ride was adapted from one I took with Sarah Clark Stuart, Campaign Director of the Bicycle Coalition of Greater Philadelphia.

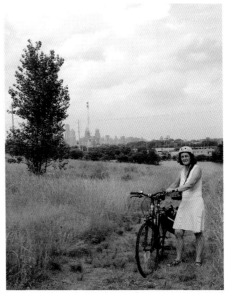

Sarah standing on the site of the new Bartram's trail.

Bartram's Garden is America's oldest living botanic garden, with a list of visitors including George Washington, Ben Franklin, and Thomas Jefferson. The 45 acre garden includes the Bartram House, meadow, parkland and wetland. The grounds are open daily until dusk.

A word to the wise – while trolley tracks, broken glass, and double parked cars are all over the city, there is a higher proportion of these obstacles on the way to Bartram's than on most other rides in this guide. So if you're not terribly comfortable riding with said conditions, this ride might not be the best for you. If you do not wish to pedal all the way to Bartram's, there is an early turn around at 43rd Street after Woodlands Cemetery. This alternate route will pick up the ride log at mile 5.4 and send you on your way back towards the Art Museum.

The route is a mix of bike path and on-road. It takes advantage of the Spring Garden bike lanes, the lesser known West Bank Greenway, and the Woodland Avenue bike lanes.

You will ride through a number of university campuses including Drexel, Upenn, and the University of the Sciences. As would be expected with a small town of college students, the food trucks in this neighborhood are some of the best in the city. If not an adventurous eater, there is a website dedicated to finding the best one for you – pennfoodtrucks.com.

The loop around Woodlands Cemetery is amazingly serene for its location in the middle of West Philadelphia. A few of the famous names buried here include Thomas Eakins, Anthony Joseph Drexel, and Edward T. Stotesbury. Have a look around – it's a cool little nook.

Sarah Clark Stuart of the Bicycle Coalition of Greater Philadelphia introduced me to the route from the Art Museum to Bartram's. The Bicycle Coalition gets a ton of results for cyclists in our region. In February 2010, Philadelphia secured $17.2 million in federal funding from the TIGER grant to build seven additional trail sections, including a new trail through Bartram's Garden, and the 58th Street Connector between Bartram's and The Cobbs Creek Recreation Path (Ride 16).

Ride Log

0.0 Start on Spring Garden bike lanes behind the Art Museum, and cross over bridge into West Philly.

0.3 Move across traffic to the left and make a left onto the 31st St bike path. Thirty-first St is one way, and this will appear to be a turn into oncoming traffic, but there is a path on the sidewalk.

0.4 Follow the bike path around the Philadelphia Boys Choir Building.

0.5 Exit path at 32nd and Powelton. Make a left onto 32nd St.

0.7 Make a right onto Arch St.

0.8 Make a left onto 34th St and pick up the bike lanes.

1.4 Right on Spruce St bike lanes.

1.9 Left on 40th St. Cross Baltimore Ave and the trolley stop.

2.1 Right on Woodland Ave bike lanes. The entrance to Woodland Cemetery is on your left.

2.4 If you wish to return at this point, make a left onto 43rd St, and pick up directions below at marker 5.4. Otherwise, continue on Woodland Ave bike lanes to 54th St.

3.4 Make a left onto 54th St. You've gone too far if you've hit 55th St.

3.6 Right on Lindberg Blvd, which forms a T in the road.

3.7 Sharp left on Harley Ave/53rd St. You've gone too far if you pass 54th or 56th St. On Harley Ave/53rd St, you'll pass Bartram's Village on the right. Follow signs towards Bartram's Garden, which is straight ahead.

3.9 Bike parking at entrance to Bartram's Garden. You're here!

 P1 East Coast Greenway
P2 WXPN Public Radio
P3 Sansom Row
P4 Penn Museum of Archaeology and Anthropology
P5 Neighborhood Bike Works, 3916 Locust Walk

 B1 Trophy Bikes, 3131 Walnut Street
B2 EMS, 3401 Chestnut St
B3 Doctor Cycles, 3608 Lancaster Ave

When ready to leave...

3.9 Exit Bartram's Garden via 53rd St/Harley Ave.

4.1 Sharp right on Lindberg Blvd.

4.2 Left on 54th St.

4.5 Right on Woodland Ave bike lanes.

5.4 Left on 43rd St.

5.8 Right on Spruce St bike lanes. If you pass Locust, you've gone too far. At Pine St, you haven't gone far enough!

6.3 Left on 38th St bike lanes.

6.6 Right on Chestnut.

7.0 Left on 33rd St.

7.4 Right on Cherry St (after Arch, before Race).

7.5 Left on 32nd St.

7.6 Make a right on 32nd and Powelton to enter bike path.

7.8 Right on Spring Garden bike lanes, over the bridge and back to the Art Museum.

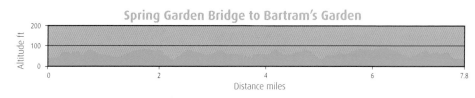

Spring Garden Bridge to Bartram's Garden

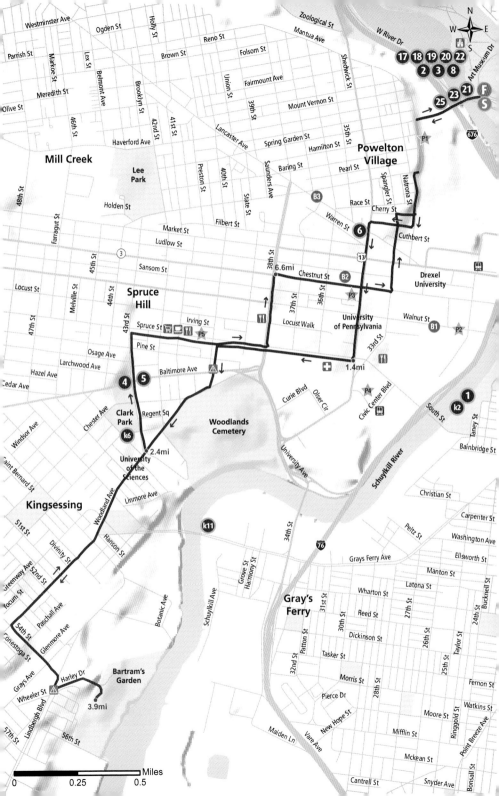

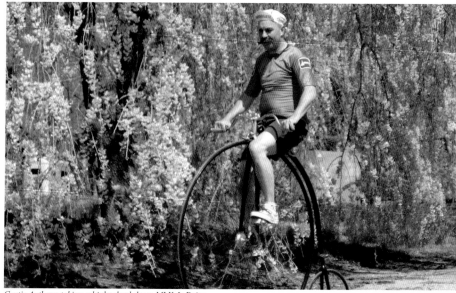

Curtis Anthony taking a high wheel down MLK Jr Drive.

At a Glance

Distance 4.6 miles   **Total Elevation** 89 feet

Terrain

This is a mix of path and bicycle lanes, with the exception of the area around Girard Avenue. There are some hilly portions close to the zoo and in East Fairmount Park.

Traffic

There is steady traffic around the zoo entrance, and a hairy intersection between 34th and Girard, but otherwise you'll be on a bike path or in cozy bike lanes.

How to Get There

The log begins at the bottom of Schuylkill Banks Park (Ride 3), on the corner of 25th and Locust. Septa buses 7, 12, and 40 will drop you nearby.

Food and Drink

A new lunch spot just opened up along Boathouse Row called Cosmic Foods. This welcomed addition sits at

the top of the row in Lloyd Hall.

Side Trip

The zoo! If you haven't been in years, then you should take this ride and spend the afternoon there. It's the first zoo in America, and there are over 1300 animals. In season (March – October), the zoo is open every day from 9:30am to 5:00pm.

Links to ❶ ❷ ❸ ❹ ❺ ❻ ❽ ⑰ ⑱ ⑲ ⑳ ㉑ ㉒ ㉓ ㉔

Where to Bike Rating 🚲🚲

About...

This short loop was suggested by Andy Dyson, former head of Neighborhood Bike Works (NBW). It was a favorite of his, and he was very enthusiastic about the portion of the East Coast Greenway in the middle of the ride. Dyson would bike there with NBW and visit the zoo in a big group; so, for the most fun possible, he and I both suggest you grab a few friends and make an afternoon out of it.

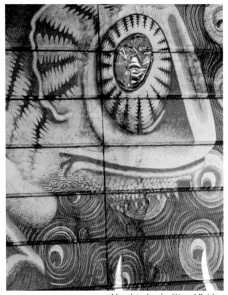

Mural under the Girard Bridge.

This one is short and sweet. You might like it if you are tired of the usual Loop (Ride 17) and you want to try a little something different.

The zoo loop begins at Schuylkill Banks Park (Ride 3), but, instead of picking up MLK Drive or continuing along the loop, you'll cross Ben Franklin Parkway and take the zigzag ramp up to Spring Garden behind the Art Museum. Cross Spring Garden at the light and take the bridge's bicycle lanes over the river and into West Philly.

Once over the river, you'll take the bike path on 31st Street towards the zoo. Part of the East Coast Greenway, this path is far less traveled than some others in the city. It will become Mantua Avenue, and then curve around to meet 34th Street.

You'll encounter traffic on 34th Street, especially as you get closer to the zoo and Girard Avenue. There's also a steep downhill here, so take it slow. The zoo will be on your left.

To return home, you'll pedal up to Girard Avenue and take the bridge over the river back into East Fairmount Park (the sidewalk on the Girard Avenue bridge is very wide). You'll make a right to pick up a series of bicycle lanes, then make a couple of turns around Sedgely and Lemon Hill to head back down to Boathouse Row.

Wait for the light to cross Kelly Drive, and make a left at Lloyd Hall to hop back on the SRT. After passing the Art Museum and the waterworks, you'll soon be riding back along the Schuylkill Banks Park towards 25th and Locust.

For more about Neighborhood Bikes Works, locations and programs, check out www.neighborhoodbikeworks.org/.

Ride Log

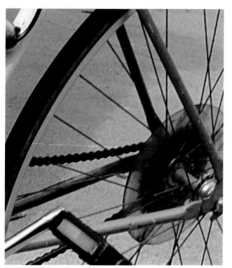

Lee's city bike.

 P1 Spring Garden Ramp
P2 The Philadelphia Zoo
P3 Lemon Hill

 B1 Trophy Bikes, 3131 Walnut St #D
B2 Volpe Cycles, 115 South 2nd St

0.0 Start at the Locust St Crossing at Schuylkill Banks Park (Ride 3) and head north.

0.1 Pass under the Walnut St Bridge.

0.6 Pass Race St entrance.

1.1 Exit the path and cross Ben Franklin Pkwy at the stoplight. You'll see a zigzag ramp that leads to Spring Garden Stand and the Art Museum just after the street. Head up the ramp!

1.2 Hop on Spring Garden bike lanes and make a left to cross the bridge over the river.

1.4 Make a right on 31st St and take the bicycle path on the right of the road – this is part of the East Coast Greenway! The path will curve around, become Mantua St, and eventually meet 34th St.

1.8 Make a right on 34th St. Check out the mural on the bridge over the railroad tracks! There's a long, straight downhill here all the way to Girard. Watch for traffic merging from I76 at the bottom of the hill.

2.4 If you have the confidence, then get in the left lane and make a left turn to the zoo entrance. If you want a more relaxing way of making the turn, then hop off your bike at Girard Ave and make a pedestrian turn.

Coming home –

2.5 After you exit the zoo, make a right on Girard to cross the Girard Bridge back to the east side of the Schuylkill.

2.6 Make the first right turn after the bridge onto Sedgley Dr.

2.8 Pass Lemon Hill.

3.0 Merge with Poplar Dr to pick up the bicycle lane. Head down the hill all the way to Kelly Dr.

3.1 Cross Kelly Dr and make a left at Lloyd Hall. You'll be heading towards the Art Museum on your way back to Schuylkill Banks Park.

3.2 Pedal alongside the old waterworks.

4.0 Pass the Race St entrance.

4.5 Pass under Walnut St Bridge.

4.6 Arrive back at Locust St entrance.

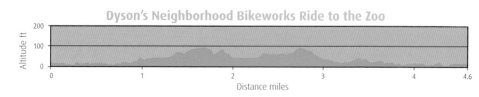

Dyson's Neighborhood Bikeworks Ride to the Zoo

Altitude ft · Distance miles

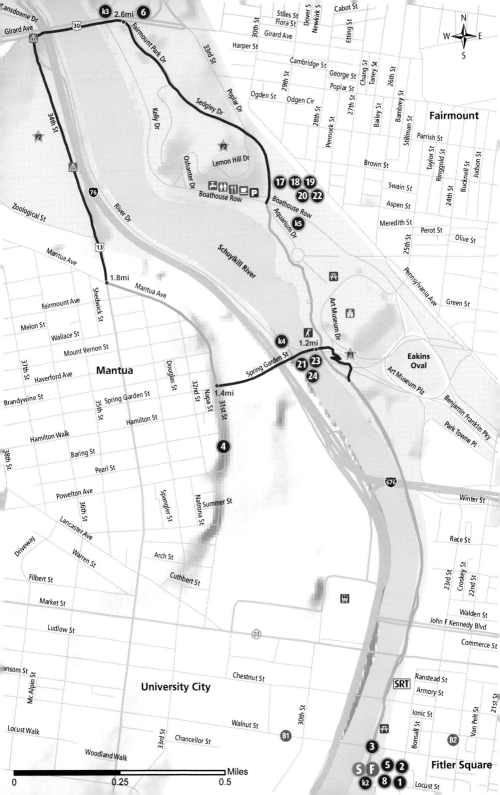

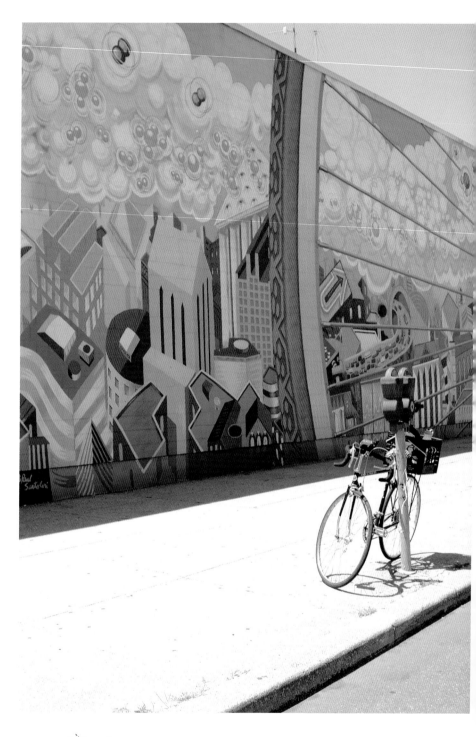

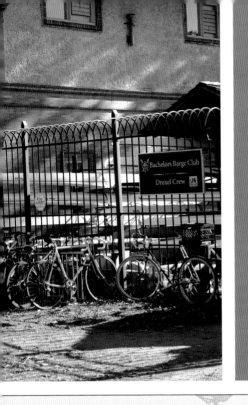
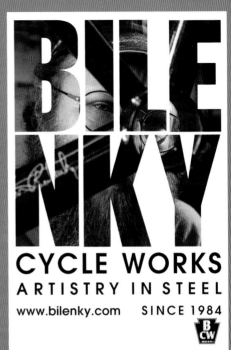

Bucks & Montgomery Counties

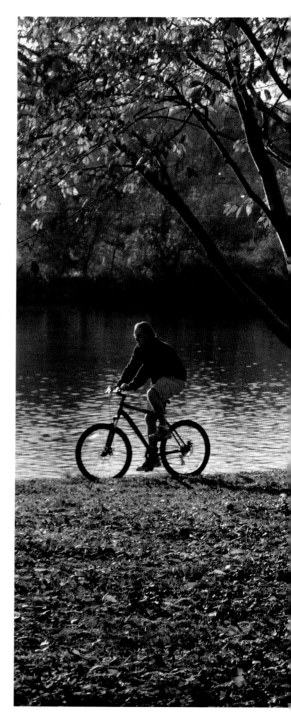

Long, hilly on-road rides and short jaunts through quiet parks on paved paths make up the majority of the routes through Bucks and Montgomery counties.

A number of these rides are excellent if you are just getting back into cycling and want to show your stuff on either car-free paths or quiet roads. And there are a ton of Regional Rail stations speckled throughout the routes – extra insurance against a mechanical problem or in the event of total poop-out! In fact, two of the rides – Jenkintown Train Station Loop (Ride 32) and the Doylestown "Bike for Barak" Loop (Ride 34) – begin and end at Regional Rail stations.

One special highlight is Ride 31 through Tyler State Park. Great for kids and families, this park is simply beautiful and the trails are very well maintained. Pedal through the lush cornstalks in the summer or the gorgeous foliage in the fall, but either way, try to get yourself and your bike out here.

If you want to ride for a long afternoon, try taking one of the Art Museum Departures to another starting point in this section. A big cycling hot spot is Bruno's in Chestnut Hill – go ahead and take Ride 20 from the city out to Bruno's, then pick up Ride 30 from Chestnut Hill to Bryn Athyn for 60 miles. This loop swings through Jenkintown and crosses Ride 32 for still more mileage.

So have fun, push your endurance, and hop on a train home if you have a bad day!

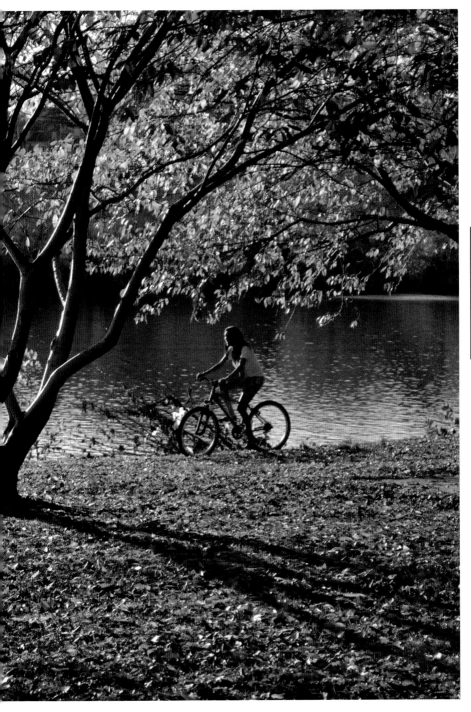

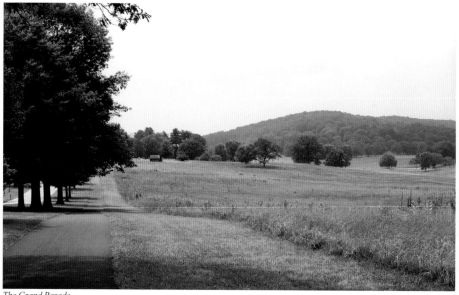

The Grand Parade.

At a Glance

Distance 5.0 miles   **Total Elevation** 259 feet

Terrain

The ride through Valley Forge follows a narrow, paved path that winds through open space, a few wooded areas, and monuments to the American Revolution.

Traffic

The paved path can have heavy bicycle and pedestrian traffic on weekends. Some cyclists prefer the tour roads that run alongside sections of the path.

How to Get There

You have a few options, my favorite being the Norristown/Manayunk line to Norristown Transportation Center (and then bike the four-ish miles on the Schuylkill River Trail to Valley Forge; the park is just over the Schuylkill River and up the hill to the left). Septa bus routes 125 and 139 stop near the visitor center, where there is also plenty of parking.

Food and Drink

The Washington Memorial Chapel, towards the end of this ride, operates a small cantina called the Cabin Shop. It's open daily from 10 to 5, and it sells cold drinks, baked goods, and even better: kitschy colonial souvenirs.

Side Trip

Pick up a Valley Forge National Park self tour brochure, produced by the U.S. Department of Interior. It will provide you with much more detailed information regarding the history of the park, and help you to understand the significance of its many monuments.

Links to   19   27   28

Where to Bike Rating

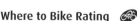

About...

The site of the 1777-1778 winter encampment of Washington's army, Valley Forge National Historical Park is a living monument to the American Revolutionary War. It pours an overwhelming sense of pride and patriotism into its visitors through pure osmosis. There are over 20 miles of trails (some paved, some packed gravel) open to bicycles in the park. The five mile route outlined here goes through the more popular areas, but you should feel free to explore as many of the trails as you wish.

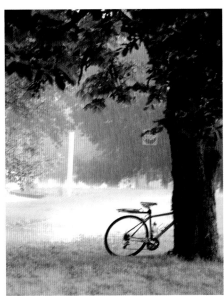

Whoops caught in the rain!

You'll start out near the visitor center – be sure to stop in and pick up some additional literature about the monuments you'll pass along the way. Heading southwest on the bike path next to Outer Line Gulph Road, you'll first pass six replica huts that stand where General Muhlenberg held the outer line of defense. Hello! There are often men dressed as colonial soldiers milling about here.

Soon you'll see the National Memorial Arch, the largest monument in the park. It stands in remembrance of the "patience and fidelity" of the soldiers who stayed in Valley Forge that winter. For an even greater dose of patriotism, hop off your bicycle and take a deep breath under the arch.

Back on your bike and full of pride, you'll follow the bike path around the arch towards Wayne's Woods. This section of the path runs adjacent to South Outer Line Drive. Before coming to the Joseph Plumb Martin Trail. (An interesting sidenote – Plumb Martin published his firsthand account of the American Revolution in 1830.) This trail follows the curves of the North Inner Line Drive.

At the top of the Plumb Martin Trail, you'll pass Varnum's Quarters, the von Steuben Statue, and the Washington Memorial Chapel, an Episopal Church built in honor of George Washington. There are regular tours of the chapel, if interested. At the very least, you should stop into the chapel's Cabin Shop for a slice of their famous "shoo-fly cake". This section of the path is next to the busy Route 23.

The downhill after the chapel is so long and so fun! Depending on your skill level, you may feel more comfortable taking the adjacent road, Route 23, down the hill. Once safely at the bottom, you'll climb a short incline up the path back to the visitor center.

If interested, there are a few shaded picnic areas in Valley Forge – Wayne's Woods, Varnum, and Betzwood.

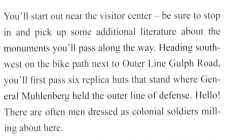

Ride Log

0.0 Hop on the trail just behind the visitor center and head south west on North Outer Line Dr.

0.3 Pass a group of log cabins to the right, marking the location of the outer line defenses. Continue along the path.

0.9 You'll see the National Memorial Arch just ahead. Bear to the right and loop around the monument. Cross Gulph Rd.

1.3 After the arch, follow the curve in the trail to the right. The road to your left is South Outer Line Dr, a one way that you should feel comfortable utilizing if the trail is too busy.

1.6 Continue to pedal along the path by making a right at the picnic area. Follow the path around Wayne's Woods.

1.8 The path becomes the Joseph Plumb Martin Trail. Watch for uneven surfaces here.

2.2 At the intersection, you'll follow the signs towards Rt 23. Go up the hill.

2.7 Cross Gulph Rd again.

3.2 Pass Varnum's Quarters and the von Steuben statue. The path runs next to the busy Rt 23. There's an awesome downhill, sometimes with deer standing in the middle! Ring your bell for the deer.

3.8 Washington Memorial Chapel is just across the street; The Cabin Shop next door has baked goods and cold drinks.

4.2 Fly down this hill!

4.6 Follow the path to the right to go back up the hill, which will bring you to your start point.

5.0 Finish at the visitor center.

P1 National Memorial Arch
P2 Varnum's Quarters
P3 Washington Memorial Chapel
P4 Grand Parade

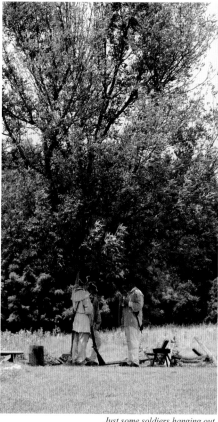

Just some soldiers hanging out.

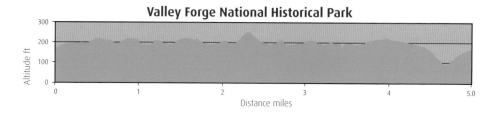

Valley Forge National Historical Park

Altitude ft

Distance miles

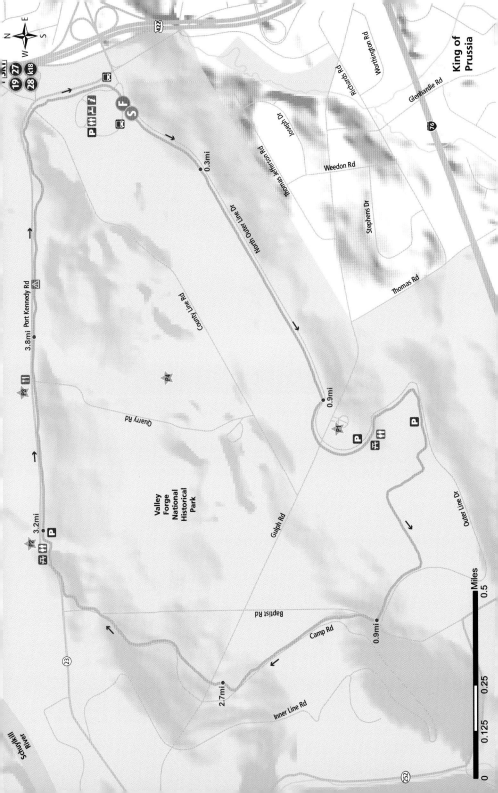

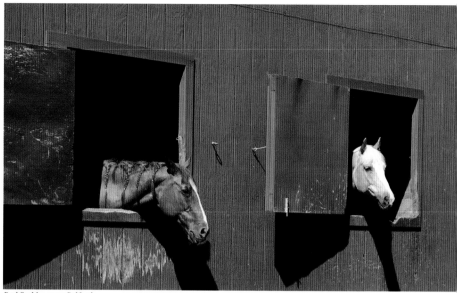

Red Stables near Salford.

At a Glance

Distance 26.4 miles   **Total Elevation** 410 feet

Terrain

The route is mostly packed gravel, with a small paved portion at the start. There will be about seven miles of on-road pedaling if you ride all the way to East Greenville.

Traffic

You are going to pass cyclists, joggers, and plenty of afternoon strollers, but the Perki trail is definitely less traveled than the SRT.

How to Get There

The ride begins on the Valley Forge section of the Schuylkill River Trail. You can park near the Betzwood picnic area just off the SRT, (about five minutes from the interchange of Route 422 and 202) or you can bike from the city to Valley Forge (Ride 19) for a 95 mile ride round trip. Septa buses 125 and 139 will bring you to Valley Forge/King of Prussia.

Food and Drink

Between miles 13 and 14, you'll pass a sweet ice cream oasis in a sea of trees and gravel; Moccia's Ice Cream Junction. The root beer floats are tops!

Side Trip

One of the best flea markets around! On Monday mornings the Perkiomenville Flea Market offers antiques, furniture and collectables, and there are over 300 dealers every week. If you pedal all the way to East Greenville, then catch a movie at The Grand – a recently restored one screen theater.

Links to **19** **26** **28**

Where to Bike Rating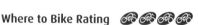

About...

The Perkiomen Trail follows the former rail bed from Valley Forge to Collegeville, Schwenksville, Salford, and Perkiomenville. This path is great in bits and pieces, but you could also pedal all the way from Philadelphia to make a weekend out of it by camping near the flea market in Perkiomenville or spending the night at The Globe Inn in East Greenville. It is about 95 miles round trip from Philadelphia to East Greenville, so be sure to bring a pal you like!

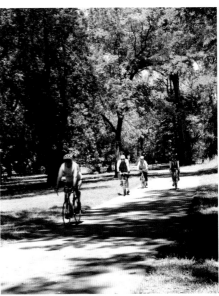

Riding through Lower Perkiomen Park.

Bring a lunch, plenty of water and extra tubes for the ride from Valley Forge to Perkiomenville. The route is a mix of on-road, paved path, and packed gravel, so choosing which bike to ride will likely take more effort than the ride itself. I went with a pal who took a durable single speed, but I brought a lighter weight road bike.

As you leave Valley Forge National Historical Park, you'll first ride through the Lower Perkiomen Valley Park and follow the luscious curves of the Perkiomen Creek for most of the ride. After you come to Upper Indian Head Road at about mile four, the trail becomes packed gravel and winds in and out of the woods. The 'out' meaning that the trail will be interrupted by a few busy streets around Collegeville – just remember there's no shame in hopping off your bike and walking across at the stoplights! The trail will pick up on the other side of these streets, and you'll be back in the woods in no time.

Otherwise, the trail is pretty well marked, and it is fairly difficult to get lost.

You'll definitely want to make an ice cream stop at Moccia's in Schwenksville, which greets you on the trail as you pass through the center of town to your left. There is always a line here in the summer and fall.

You'll come to a pretty steep downhill around mile 14. It's a lot of fun to take, but can lead to a nice wipe-out or two because of the packed gravel. You may feel some anxiety about climbing this beast on your way home; just knock that gear down and let your tires spin as you climb back up.

The flat gravel path comes to an end on Upper Ridge Road, though I recently caught wind of a single track extension through Green Lane Park. If you are chugging out to East Greenville, then your best bet is Route 29. It can be busy, but by this stage of the ride, you'll be so ready to get off your bike that you'll totally burn it up! Just remember, before you hit East Greenville the street numbers go down and then back up – you want the second Fourth Street if you're heading to The Globe.

Ride 27 - Valley Forge to Perkiomenville

Ride Log

0.0 Start on the Schuylkill River Trail at Valley Forge, heading west.

1.1 Stay on the SRT, exit Valley Forge National Historical Park.

1.7 Cross the bridge and follow the switchback.

1.9 You'll come to the Phonexville/Perkiomen/SRT trail junction. Make a left to pedal towards the Perkiomen Trail. Ride through the Lower Perkiomen Valley Park.

3.9 Left on Upper Indian Head Rd.

4.1 Right to enter the Perki Trail (this is packed gravel). You are going to follow this for many, many miles!

7.3 The trail pops you out on Second Ave in Collegeville. There is a drugstore on the corner if you need a cold drink or granola bar. Cross Second Ave and pick up the trail alongside the drugstore.

7.7 The trail pops out, again, on the street. The Collegeville Diner is on the corner. Cross Third Ave, make a right on Ridge Park and then a left to pick up the trail (Pooped? The 93 bus will take you to Norristown Transportation Center).

8.7 One more time! Cross Rt 29 and pick up the Perki path on the other side.

10.5 Ride over the bridge to cross the Perkiomen Creek. This is a nice spot to cool off and dunk your feet.

13.3 Pass Tailwind Bicycles to the left of the trail. You're in Schwenksville!

13.5 Moccias Ice Cream…Yes.

P1 Perkiomenville Flea Market
P2 The Grand Theater,
    252 Main St, East Greenville
P3 The Globe Inn, 326 West 4th St

B1 The Bike Shop
    1987 West Main St, Eagleville
B2 Bikesport
    325 West Main St, Collegeville
B3 Tailwind Bicycles
    160 Main St, Schwenksville

13.7 Cross Schwenksville Rd and follow the path – it will curve right and then left. Follow the path back through the wooded area.

14.5 Twelve percent downhill!

15.0 Cross Spring Mt Rd and pick up trail.

16.7 Cruisin' through Salford.

19.6 Come to Upper Ridge Rd and Rt 29. You've reached Perkiomenville! The flea market happens on this corner every Monday. There is camping nearby as well. If you are heading all the way to East Greenville, you'll hop on Rt 29 and follow signs north.

20.8 One of the first of a few hills on the way to East Greenville.

21.8 Oh boy, there's another.

22.3 OUCH, there is the third hill!

25.7 Rt 29 becomes Main St. The street numbers wind down to First/Front St, and then go up again.

26.2 Left on Fourth St.

26.4 Arrive at The Globe Inn.

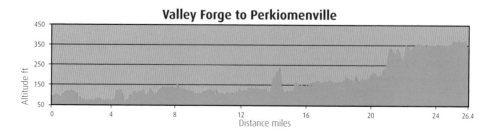

Valley Forge to Perkiomenville

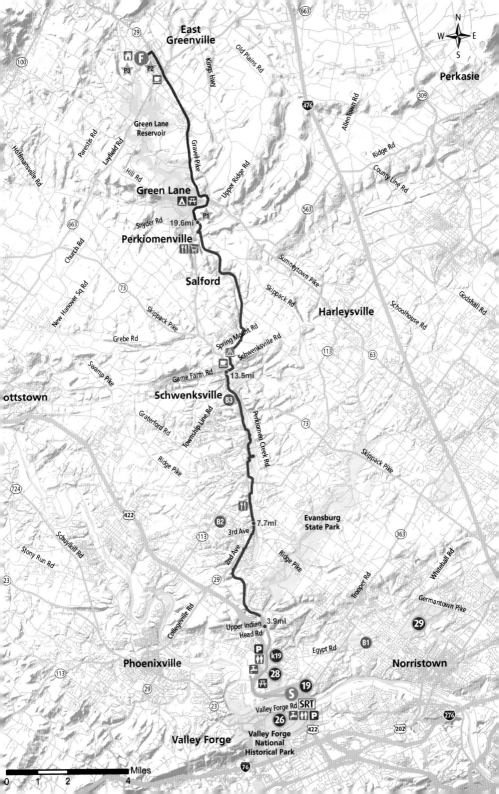

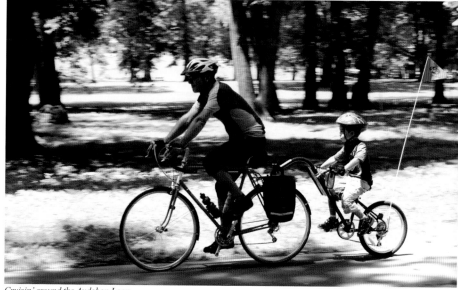

Cruisin' around the Audobon Loop.

At a Glance

Distance 4.1 miles   **Total Elevation** 207 feet

Terrain

A paved path running alongside secluded wooded areas, bird sanctuaries, and a creek.

Traffic

The Audubon Loop generally has less bicycle and pedestrian traffic than its friend across the way, the Valley Forge National Historic Park.

How to Get There

The best mode of travel to Audubon Loop is your bicycle! It meets the Schuylkill River Trail at Valley Forge (Ride 19) and the start of the Perkiomen Trail (Ride 27). Of course if you have to drive, you'll find parking at the Pawlings Road trail head.

Food and Drink

A few water fountains welcome you to the Lower Perkiomen Valley Park, but, if you intend to stay on the loop, then plan to bring some snacks for a picnic.

Side Trip

The John James Audubon Center at Mill Grove! Audubon's first home in the United States, the 175 acre site is listed on the National Register of Historic Places. The museum houses the famous *Birds of America* collection, among much of Audubon's other artwork and writings. Admission is a steal at $4 for adults.

Links to

Where to Bike Rating

About...

The Audubon Loop takes you through the Lower Perkiomen Valley Park and, as the name implies, the John James Audubon Center at Mill Grove. Mostly flat save for a couple of hills (including one nine percent grade incline), the loop is an excellent four mile addition to an afternoon ride on the Schuylkill River Trail. Of course, it also stands alone if you wish to explore the museum or some of the Audubon bird sanctuaries.

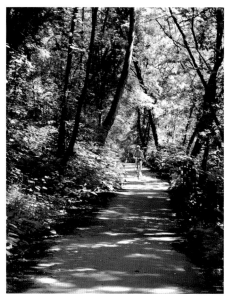

She went counter clockwise.

Hop on your bicycle and let your mind wander…what did John James Audubon see here 200 years ago? These woods were a thrilling playground for the young artist, author, and naturalist.

The ride log takes you counter clockwise – certainly the easier route. If you are looking for a better challenge or some practice with hills, reverse the directions to ride clockwise.

You'll start out at the intersection between the SRT, the Perkiomen Trail, and the Audubon Loop. To go the easy way, head up the switchback towards Pawlings Road. To tackle the more challenging route, pedal straight ahead – towards the Lower Perkiomen Valley Park (Ride K18).

Assuming, like me, you do not wish to climb a nine percent grade, then you have picked the easy way towards Pawlings Road. From here you will make a left over the bridge and follow Audubon Loop (marked on the path itself as 'AL'). You'll travel alongside Pawlings Road for about a mile, passing a few bird observation areas and eventually the John James Audubon Center at Mill Grove (1201 Pawlings Road). The sanctuary grounds are open from 7am until dusk.

After the left at Audubon Road, you'll soon pass a smoke stack that dates back to the mid-19th century copper and lead ore mining activities at Mill Grove. The sign near the stack notes that over 1,500 tons of lead was mined in here between 1813 and 1825!

You'll hit the steep grade and continue to follow the path until Egypt Road. The path becomes an awkward sidewalk along the bridge. Follow the sidewalk over the bridge and make a left afterwards. The sidewalk ends, but there will be a barrier between you and the road to make you feel secure. The entrance to the Lower Perkiomen Valley Park can be easy to miss – look for the red sign and parking lot. Once back on the path, you'll take a right to pedal through the park (or, take a left to pick up Ride 27). Stop here for a drink at the water fountains or a quick game of tetherball.

When you leave the park, you'll come to a fork. Bear right to pick up the Schuylkill River Trail (the pavement will be painted 'SRT') and follow the switchback over the bridge. Continue straight and you'll find yourself at the familiar Pawlings Road switchback. Bear right to head towards the parking lot, left to head towards Valley Forge.

Ride Log

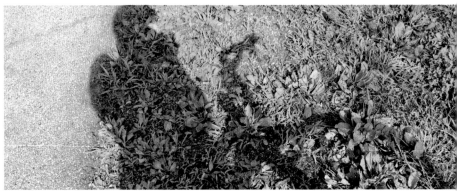

Late afternoon shadows.

* If coming from Valley Forge on the Schuylkill River Trail (SRT), follow the signs towards Pawlings Rd.

0.0 If coming from SRT, make a left at the Pawlings switchback and head up the path.

0.2 Pass the trailhead parking lot to your right, and make a left to follow 'AL' (Audubon Loop) over the bridge. The path runs alongside Pawlings Rd.

0.8 Pass a lovely bird watching area, part of the Audubon Wildlife Sanctuary. Follow the trail into the trees.

1.1 Cross Old Mill Rd and climb up a short, steep hill.

1.3 Pass the John James Audubon Center at Mill Grove. Bear left to follow the path at the corner of Pawlings and Audubon.

1.4 Follow the trail through the woods!

1.8 Pass the Mill Grove smoke stack, dating back to 1855.

1.9 Enjoy the nine percent grade downhill – Wheeeeeeeeeeeee!

2.2 The path pops out onto Egypt Rd. Make a left and

P1 John James Audubon Center, 1201 Pawlings Rd, Mill Grove
P2 Audubon Wildlife Sanctuary

follow the sidewalk/path over the bridge.

2.4 The sidewalk/path ends after the bridge. Hook a left after the bridge on New Mill Rd.

2.5 Make another left to enter the Lower Perkiomen Valley Park. At the entrance, make a right to pick up the Perkiomen Trail.

3.2 The trail begins to follow the Perkiomen Creek to your left. There is an excellent picnic area with BBQs and tetherball just ahead.

3.7 Bear right to head up the switchback. Follow signs for Schuylkill River Trail, or SRT (which is painted on the pavement along with an arrow).

3.9 Over the bridge.

4.1 Arrive at the bottom of the Pawlings Rd switchback.

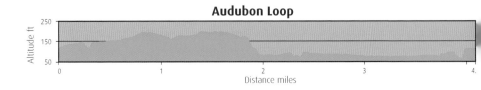

Audubon Loop

Altitude ft

Distance miles

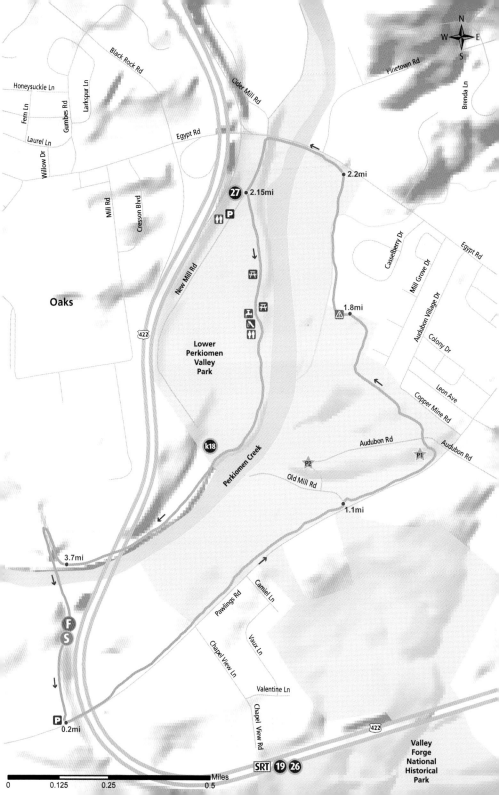

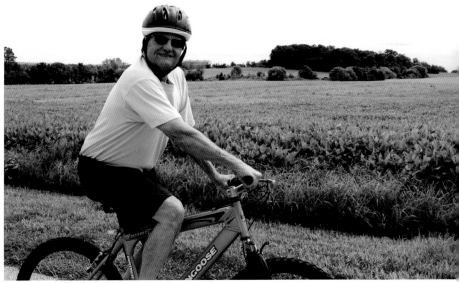

Cruising around Norristown Farm Park.

At a Glance

Distance 5.4 miles   **Total Elevation** 265 feet

Terrain
You'll be riding on a paved path that goes up and down, and up, and up and down again. Some portions might benefit from a bit of resurfacing.

Traffic
The usual bike/ped crowd will accompany you through the farm park, though it is less traveled than some of the other bike paths in the area. I also think there are a lot of ghosts roaming the land.

How to Get There
From the Norristown Transportation Center, take Farm Park Route A (Haws Avenue/Stanbridge Street) just off of the Schuylkill River Trail (mile 16.4 on Ride 19). If you're not keen on riding through Norristown, then your best bet is to drive and park at the Whitehall Road parking lot.

Food and Drink
BYOP - Bring Your Own Picnic!

Side Trip
Did you know there was a zoo in Norristown? Me neither! The Elmwood Zoo, located nearby at 1661 Harding Boulevard, has sat on this corner since 1924. There are exhibits on wetlands, woodlands, and bayou, among others. They also offer the popular Zoosnooze (a terrifically named sleepover!) in the summer.

Links to

Where to Bike Rating

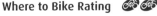

About...

There are eight miles of jumbled trails traversing Norristown Farm Park's 690 acres, a stunning backdrop for getting turned about in a hodgepodge of trails. Fifteen historic buildings dot the park, the oldest of which dates back to the mid 18th century. The land has been a working farm for over 200 years, and provides, in this author's opinion, a setting for a bicycle ride that is both spooky and oddly alluring.

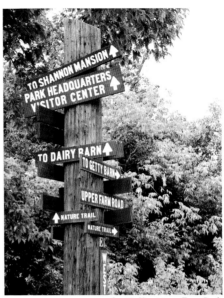

Lost in Norristown Farm Park.

Bucks & Montgomery Counties

A disclaimer: I visited the Norristown Farm Park on a cloudy afternoon. It happened to be Friday the 13th, and found the place, well, creepy. What are all of these boarded up old barns and buildings? What is the deal with Norristown State Hospital right next door? Wait, there is a zoo around the block? I'd bet that the park would be more inviting on a sunny day!

The bridges and rolling hills make for an interesting ride through the farm park, as does the unusual setting - it is a working farm (450 acres are still tilled every year) next to a mental health facility, Norristown State Hospital, in the middle of a fairly urban area. Until 1975, patients at the hospital worked on the farm as it was believed to improve recovery. There are old railroad tracks, a cemetery, boarded historical buildings (that look less inviting than even Norristown State) next to creeks, ponds and a trout nursery, 263 species of wildflowers and 73 species of birds.

You'll start out at the Whitehall Road parking lot, simply because it is the easiest to find. You'll arrive at intersection after intersection of trails, some with decent signage (the first turn towards the dairy barn, for example, is well marked), and some where there's no way to tell whether you are on a path, a trail, or a road.

There are also a lot of surprising dead ends!

The park office is near the dairy barn, as is an additional parking lot. If you start out here, then simply pick up the ride log at mile 1.2. You can acquire a fairly confusing map of the farm park, published by the PA Department of Conservation and Natural Resources, at the park office or at the Whitehall trail head.

The Doctors House at mile 2.3 and the Happy Hollow Cottage a mile 3.9 would play perfect host as spooky haunted houses.

There is an on-road connector to the Schuylkill River Trail at Stainbridge Road that connects to Haws Avenue and takes you through Norristown.

There's quite a bit of history at Norristown Farm Park. If you'd like to learn more about the sale of the land from William Penn to Isaac Norris in 1704, the five plantations that sprung up in the 18th century, or current preservation initiatives, visit The Farm Park Preservation Association at www.farmpark.org.

Ride Log

0.0 Start out at the Whitehall Rd parking lot, and make a left on the path.

0.6 When you reach the bottom of the hill, make a left at the stop sign. Follow arrows towards the dairy barn.

0.7 After the bridge, bear left to pick up the small path that runs alongside Upper Farm Rd. Take the path into the woods. Lots of inviting picnic areas here!

1.0 Follow the path as it winds to the right.

1.2 Pass the dairy barn to your right and continue straight.

1.4 Follow the trail down the hill and make a hairpin turn. Cross Upper Farm Rd and enter the path that is closed to motor vehicles (you'll know by the many Do Not Enter signs!).

1.6 Cross the Meadow Bridge over Stony Creek (yes, those are the actual names). Follow the path to the right.

1.8 Make a left over the railroad tracks and another quick left. Make a right to head up the hill on the path.

2.1 Pass the Norris City Cemetery to the left, zoom down the hill.

2.2 Make a sharp right at the T in the path.

2.4 Make another right at the fork (if you hit a creek you've gone too far).

2.7 Come to a bridge that, at the time of writing, lies in wait to be repaired. Make one more right!

3.0 Cross the railroad tracks again, then make a left back onto the path. Follow this path for a ways.

3.5 Cross the Stanbridge St Bridge (connector to the Schuylkill River Trail is to your left, if interested). Make a right on Stony Creek Rd.

3.7 Pedal through the foot/bicycle traffic entrance.

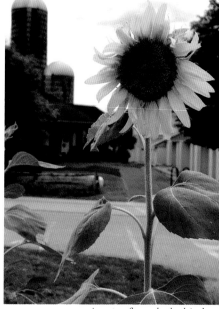

August sunflowers by the dairy barn

Continue straight.

4.0 Come to this familiar junction, and make a left back on Upper Farm Rd.

4.3 At the top of the hill, make a right to go around the old barn. Follow the path with an immediate left. Cruise down the hill ahead.

4.9 Follow the path to the right. You'll be perched on the corner of Sterigere St and Whitehall Rd.

5.4 Back at the start!

Norristown Farm Park

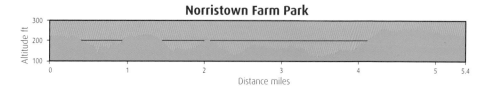

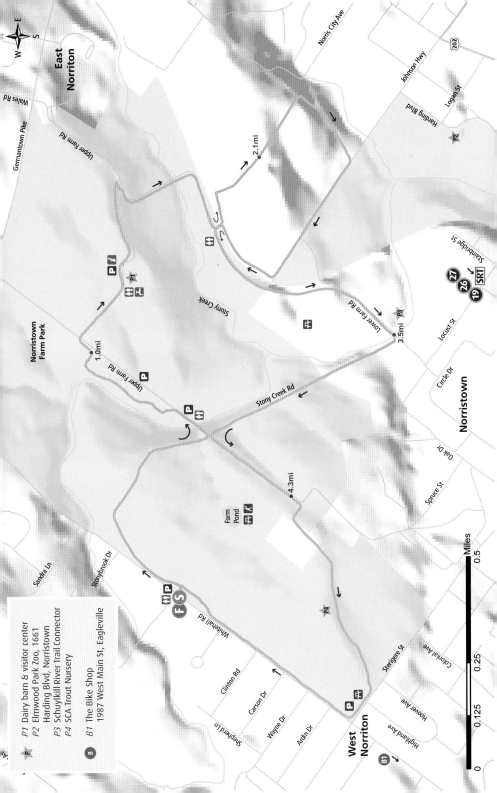

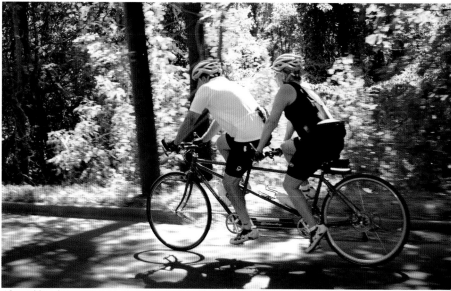

A beautiful tandem.

At a Glance

Distance 27.5 miles **Total Elevation** 423 feet

Terrain

You'll be riding on heavily cycled suburban roads that go up and down and up and down.

Traffic

There are some narrow roads along the way and a handful of busy intersections, but for the most part you will enjoy wide shoulders and residential streets.

How to Get There

Parking is located at the Forbidden Drive trailhead (Ride 12) on Northwestern Avenue. You can also take the Chestnut Hill West line to Highland Avenue and follow Ride 20 log (starting at mile marker 11.3) to ride the two miles to Bruno's. Or – follow the full Ride 20 log and pedal all the way from Center City to Bryn Athyn for a sweet 60 mile loop!

Food and Drink

Bruno's – an obvious and excellent choice – is at the start of the ride. You'll pass pockets of rest stops and snack shops every few miles, including a Whole Food around mile seven and a bunch of cafés in the heart of Jenkintown at mile 19.

Side Trip

Visit the Bryn Athyn Cathedral and stroll through the rolling hills that surround this magnificent structure constructed between 1913 and 1928.

Links to 12 13 14 20 32

Where to Bike Rating

About...

This loop is brought to you courtesy of Thomas Madle, a longtime ride leader for the Bicycle Club of Philadelphia – it's one of his absolute favorites (and now one of mine too!). You will pedal from Chestnut Hill to Jenkintown, on towards Bryn Athyn and Huntington Valley, then back in a long, luxurious loop. While there will be some busy intersections to navigate, the route is chock full of wide residential roads, rest stops, and poop-out train stations.

I went on this loop with my dad, and we were both excited about all of the cyclists we saw along the way. And with so many little hills this way and that, it is a great ride for getting the heart pumping. Be ready for the steady incline waiting for you in miles 16 through 20. The last two miles are a fun and fast downhill.

You'll see a lot of different suburbs on this loop. Starting in Chestnut Hill, you'll make your way towards Flourtown, Oreland, and Glenside. You'll go through Jenkintown on your way out to Bryn Athyn, loop around Fox Chase, then head back to Chestnut Hill via Wyncote, Cheltenham, and Wyndmoor.

The Bryn Athyn Cathedral, built between 1913 and 1928 by members of the New Church, peeks through the trees on Alnwick Road before it comes into full view. It has amazing stained glass windows and, according to its history, not a single right angle or straight line. The Bryn Athyn Historic District was designated as a National Historic Landmark in 2008 – there are daily tours if interested.

On your return, you'll pass Fox Chase Farm before eventually reaching Jenkintown (mile 19.7), another town where you might want to stop for a bite or a stroll. You'll cycle down West Avenue, home to many shops and cafés.

If you wish to increase the length of the ride, add on Ride 20 (Boathouse Row to Bruno's) or Ride 32 (Jenkintown Train Station Loop). You will also cross the entrances to Forbidden Drive in Chestnut Hill and Pennypack Park in Fox Chase – two wooded, gravel packed bikeways that make for shaded picnic stops.

A big thanks goes out to Tom Madle for this cue – these are all great roads for biking. If you like this ride, you might want to try another of his loops: Okehocking Hills (Ride 39).

Ride Log

0.0 Start out at Bruno's, on the corner of Northwestern Ave and Germantown Pike.

0.6 Cross Stenton Ave.

1.7 Three fast turns here: Right on Kopley Rd, a left on McCloskey, and a right on Chestnut Ln.

2.0 Left on Haws Ln. There will be slightly more traffic here than on the previous residential streets.

2.9 Right on Church Rd at the T.

3.3 Left on Paper Mill Rd.

3.6 Right on Edann Rd.

4.1 Left on Station Ave at the T.

4.9 Right on Mt Carmel Ave. This is a weird turn – take the sharp right.

6.1 Cross Easton Rd.

6.7 Left on Highland Ave.

6.9 Right on Wharton Rd (at the second light). Bear left towards Baeder Rd.

7.8 Left on Old York Rd, then a very fast right onto The Fairway. Caution please!

8.4 Whole Foods Market to the left for a snack.

8.5 Left on Rydal Rd, becomes Valley Rd.

11.1 Left on Terwood Rd and up the quick hill.

11.2 Right on Fetters Mill Rd.

11.5 Bear Left on Alnwick Rd.

11.8 Look left to see the Cathedral!

12.0 Cross Huntington Pike – Alnwick becomes Tomlinson Rd (you will be biking through the campus of Academy of the New Church). Follow Tomlinson past Buck Rd and Philmont Ave. There are a few zigzags as

Ride Log continued..

you bike through Philmont Country Club.

13.3 Right onto Pine Rd.

14.4 Left on Welsh Rd at the T.

14.6 Right to get back onto Pine Rd.

15.9 Cross Moredun Rd. The entrance to Pennypack Park (Ride 14) is just ahead.

16.3 Bear right to pick up Shady Ln (just past Fox Chase Farm). Shady Ln is narrow.

17.6 Right on Fox Chase Rd.

18.4 Pass Alverthorpe Park to the right.

19.0 Right on Meetinghouse Rd at the T.

19.1 Immediate left on Fair Acres.

19.4 Left on Washington Ln.

19.5 Right on Newbold Rd, and a quick left onto West Ave.

19.7 Cross Old York Rd and you're in Jenkintown! Snacks and coffee here.

20.5 Follow the left curve in the road as you come to the Jenkintown train station.

20.6 Right on Greenwood Ave to take the bridge over the train tracks.

20.7 Right onto Glenside Ave.

21.0 Left onto Waverly Rd. Stay on Waverly for about 2.5 miles. Cross Easton Rd and Limekiln Pike.

22.4 Bear left to remain on Waverly. Cross Church Rd.

23.5 Right on Cheltenham Ave.

23.8 Left on Willow Grove Ave.

24.0 Right on Douglas Rd.

24.3 Left on Churchill Rd.

24.4 Right on Southhampton Ave.

24.8 Right on Flourtown Ave at the T.

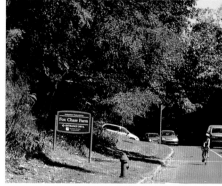
Riding past Fox Chase Farm.

25.0 Left on Gravers Ln.

25.1 Right on Ardmore Ave.

25.3 Left at Evergreen.

25.3 Right on Montgomery. There is a long awesome downhill here, with a light at the end.

26.4 Left on Bethlehem Pike.

26.5 Right on Gordon Rd.

26.8 Right on Stenton Ave.

27.0 Left on Northwestern/Wissahickon Ave.

27.5 End at Bruno's!

P1 Morris Arboretum
P2 Bryn Athyn Cathedral
P3 Fox Chase Farm

B *B1* Erdenheim Bicyle & Fitness
821 Bethlehem Pike #3, Glenside
B2 Keswick Cycle Co
408 Easton Road, Glenside
B3 Abington Wheel Wright
1120 Old York Road, Abington

Tom's Trek from Chestnut Hill to Bryn Athyn

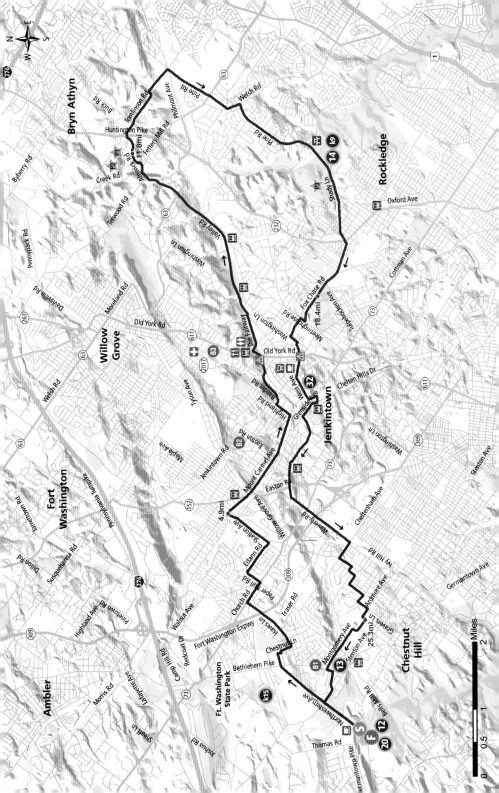

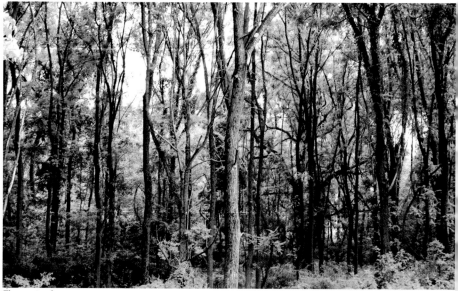

The teeming forest.

At a Glance

Distance 4.7 miles   **Total Elevation** 308 feet

Terrain

There are a lot of hills on this wide, paved trail!

Traffic

The traffic changes on every path – on some you'll pass by joggers and baby strollers, others will have horses, and a few will be blissfully empty.

How to Get There

The 130 Septa bus will drop you at Bucks County Community College, situated directly next to the park. The entrance to Tyler is a short ride down Swamp Road from Exit 49 off I-95. There are plenty of parking lots too, the largest of which is near the boat house area.

Food and Drink

In the summer, there's usually an ice cream truck hanging around the boat house area. Otherwise, a drive into Newtown (via Swamp or Richboro Road) has options for a meal or a snack.

Side Trip

You'll pass The Earth Center for the Arts on Stable Mill Trail. They offer classes, workshops, craft fairs and other community events. Just next to the center, there is a wild meadow speckled with rad outdoor art and sculpture. Upcoming events are regularly posted on their website: www.ec4ta.org.

Where to Bike Rating

About...

Tyler State Park absolutely takes the cake for my favorite off-road paved path. Between the horses, corn fields, and forests that would well suit a production of *A Midsummer's Night Dream*, cyclists are immediately transplanted to the beautiful, bucolic countryside. The terrain is varied, with lots of climbing, fast downhills and snappy curves. It is about a five mile loop, but you'll find there are plenty of additional trails to explore.

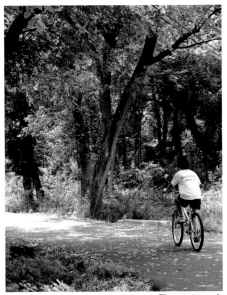

The twisting path.

In all seriousness, you have got to check out Tyler State Park. You will not be disappointed! It is as visually appealing as it is challenging, and the trails offer enough loops and track backs to explore the park weekend after weekend. The trails are well marked and expertly manicured, offering a pleasant and comfortable setting for an afternoon ride.

You'll start out near the boat house area, which is just next to the main parking area (to get here, you'll need to pick up Main Park Road and drive a ways until you reach the center of the park). Take the bridge over Neshaminy Creek, which is usually full of bathers. It is pure heaven to have a splash in the water here after you finish your ride.

The loop takes advantage of the Dairy Hill Trail, White Pine Trail, Number One Trail, Stable Mill Trail, and Natural Area Trail, which are all west of the Neshaminy Creek. The woman in the park office was fearful that I might get lost in Tyler's 1700 acres, and she assured me that I could just give them a ring and a park ranger would come pick me up (215-968-2021, should you fall into this fate).

The first mile along Dairy Hill Trail is fairly flat, but almost all of mile two is a steady climb. There are a couple of really fun and fast downhills on the Number One Lane Trail, but they are almost always immediately followed by a twisting turn, so keep it slow.

If you want an intense hill challenge, simply reverse the ride log. You'll go up some of the steeper hills and enjoy the slow downhill that you would otherwise climb between miles one and two. Explore as many trails as possible. You'll pass wooded areas, open meadows, and horse stables. Farmers sow about a quarter of the park every year – in late August the corn is teeming and simply gorgeous on a sunny afternoon.

You can also make a weekend out of it! There is a hostel at the Solly Farmhouse and Annex near the Schofield Covered Bridge, operated by Hosteling International. Other activities in the park include disk golf, fishing, sledding, ice skating, and boating. There are about a half dozen picnic areas and an entire network of equestrian trails. Go! Now!

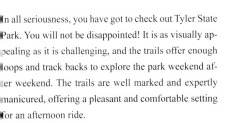

Ride Log

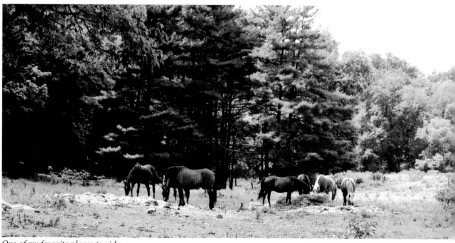

One of my favorite places to ride.

0.0 Start out by the boat house area, near the main parking lot. Cross the bridge over the Neshaminy Creek.

0.1 Make a right at the T, just past the bridge.

0.5 At Dairy Hill Trail, make a right.

0.8 Follow the trail as it curves to the left. The locusts here are so loud in the summer!

1.5 Come to an intersection with cornfields and water fountains. If you want a slight detour, make a right on the Covered Bridge Trail to visit the Schofield Covered Bridge (built in 1874, it's the longest covered bridge in Bucks County!) If you don't care about covered bridges, then pedal straight ahead towards the cornfields along the White Pine Trail.

1.9 Make a left at the stop sign to continue along White Pine Trail. Follow the sign that points you towards the boat house. Great downhill here.

2.1 Make a right to get on the Number One Ln Trail, there's a barn on the corner. Enjoy the fast downhills and sharp turns of Number One Ln.

3.1 Cross the bridge, at the intersection with College Park Trail, bear left to stay on Number One.

3.3 Stay on Number One, passing the parking lot to the right. Make a left on Stable Mill Trail (you may encounter a car here and there on this road).

3.6 You'll pass the Earth Center for the Arts on the right.

3.8 Bear left at the intersection to head towards Natural Area Trail. Another fast downhill here! Follow Natural Area Trail – beware the sharp turns!

4.6 Come to a T and make a left on Mill Dairy Trail.

4.7 Back to the bridge! Make a right to cross the bridge and head back to the boat house.

The Teeming, Twisting Tyler State Park

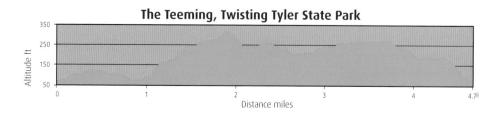

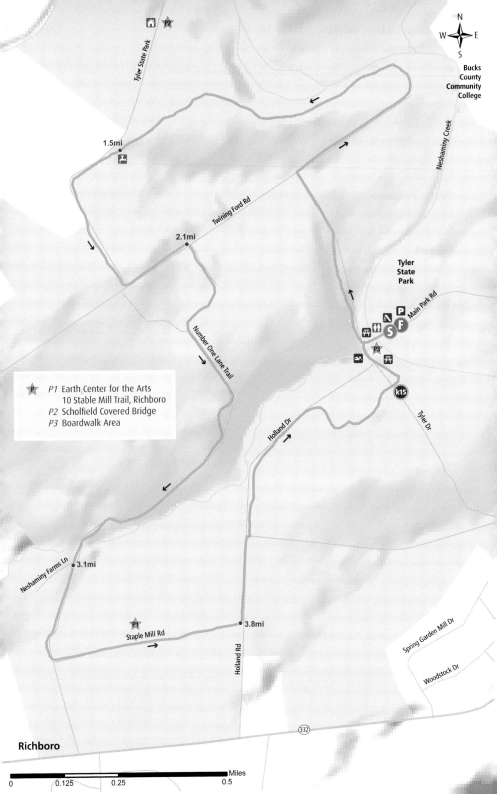

N
W · E
S

P2

Tyler State Park

Bucks County Community College

Neshaminy Creek

1.5mi

Twining Ford Rd

2.1mi

Tyler State Park

P
Main Park Rd

S F

P3

k15

Number One Lane Trail

P1 Earth Center for the Arts
10 Stable Mill Trail, Richboro
P2 Scholfield Covered Bridge
P3 Boardwalk Area

Tyler Dr

Holland Dr

3.1mi

Neshaminy Farms Ln

P1

Staple Mill Rd

3.8mi

Holland Rd

Spring Garden Mill Dr

Woodstock Dr

332

Richboro

Miles

0   0.125   0.25   0.5

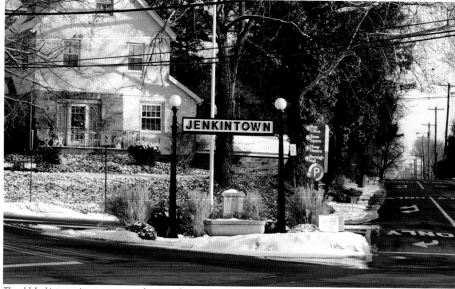

The old Jenkintown sign greets you at the start of your ride.

At a Glance

Distance 3.8 miles   **Total Elevation** 340 feet

Terrain

The quiet loop around Jenkintown mixes a few soft hills with calm, quiet streets and mostly flat terrain. You'll be cycling on road for the full trip.

Traffic

There is minimal traffic on most of these roads, with the exception of brief stints on Washington Lane and West Avenue. You'll also cross the very busy Old York Road, but you will have the help of traffic lights to keep you on your way.

How to Get There

The ride log begins at the Jenkintown train station, so grab your bike and hop on any of the following Septa lines: Landale/Doylestown, Warminster, or West Trenton. Trains run very frequently out here, but be sure to time your ride to avoid peak hours! (see You, Your Bike, and Transport in Philly for details). There is also parking at the station.

Food and Drink

You'll ride right through the center of Jenkintown, which has a number of cafés and sandwich shops, including the West Avenue Grille. The challah French toast is the obvious, excellent choice here.

Side Trip

After downing said challah French toast, visit Shakti West for a drop in yoga session. Shakti, located at West Avenue and Cedar Street, offers a variety of classes every day – call ahead to time your ride and your breakfast accordingly!

Links to

Where to Bike Rating

About...

Want to get out of the city for a short ride? Try Jenkintown on for size! The ride begins and ends at the Jenkintown train station and brings you through quiet, residential streets on your way towards the center of town. In just a few blocks along West Avenue, you can stop for lunch, see a movie, eat a cupcake in the town square, visit a thrift shop, or take a yoga class. And, you'll be finished in under four miles.

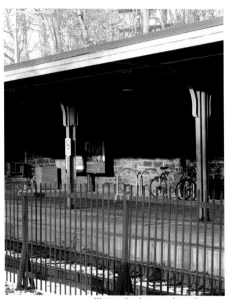

Waiting for the train, late afternoon.

Bucks & Montgomery Counties

The loop around Jenkintown is a quick vacation from the city, with quiet streets and relatively low traffic. This ride is also the perfect occasion to practice bringing your bicycle on Septa! Jenkintown is served by three different train lines, which means you'll never have to wait too long for a ride out there or back home. Pick up a copy of the Glenside Combined Schedule for more details.

From the Jenkintown train station, follow West Avenue to Runnymede. The quiet, treelined streets are ideal for relaxed riding. You'll cross Walnut Street at the light, which is a slightly busier intersection. A little farther down Runnymede and you'll hit a high traffic intersection – the corner of Starbucks and Wawa on Old York Road. Be sure to follow the traffic patterns and cross at the light.

After Old York Road, you'll climb around Rydal for a bit before coming out on Washington Lane. You won't be on Washington for very long, but it is busier than most of the other streets you'll be riding on. Make a turn back towards Jenkintown just before Abington Friends School on Vernon Road, and then a quick left onto West Avenue.

The corner of West and Old York Road is the en-trance to the center of town, which is very small and very adorable. You'll have your choice of cafés and snack shops here, including a delicious cupcake bakery and coffee shop. There are also some fun boutiques and gift shops, if so inclined. Jenkintown hosts a number of seasonal music and art festivals as well – check out www.jenkintown.net for dates and details.

There is also a terrific restored theater nearby, a one screen vintage beaut' called the Hiway. They screen independent and foreign films and always have matinees. The Hiway is located on Old York Road, two blocks south of the West Avenue intersection.

You'll ride a bit farther on West Avenue, followed by a few more suburban roads back to the train station. What a lovely afternoon!

Ride Log

0.0 Start on West Ave (the side where incoming trains from the city depart) and head north. You'll make a quick bend by the stop sign.

0.3 Left on Runnymede, follow the bend.

0.7 Cross Walnut St.

1.2 Follow the traffic laws around the circle to make your way across Old York Rd. Use caution here. Pick up Rodman Ave after you cross.

1.5 Right on Noble Rd.

1.6 Bear left at the fork on Pepper Rd.

1.9 Right on Worrell.

2.0 Left on Fairhill Rd.

2.2 Right on Gregory Rd, followed by quick right on Red Rambler Rd.

2.4 Left on Washington Ln – busier than the other roads along this route.

2.7 Right on Vernon Rd, just before Abington Friends School.

2.8 Quick left onto West Ave. Pedal through the heart of Jenkintown.

3.0 Left on Leedom St.

3.1 Right on Summit Ave.

3.6 Pop out on West Ave, make a right towards the train station.

3.8 Back to the train!

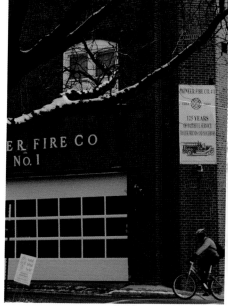

Pedaling around the firehouse.

P *P1* Jenkintown Square
P2 Shakti Yoga, 605 West Avenue, Jenkintown
P3 Hiway Theater, 212 Old York Rd, Jenkintown
P4 Abington Art Center,
515 Meetinghouse Rd, Jenkintown

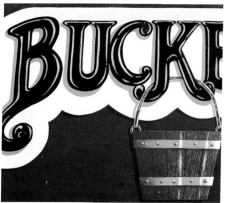

A watering hole on West Avenue.

Jenkintown Train Station Loop

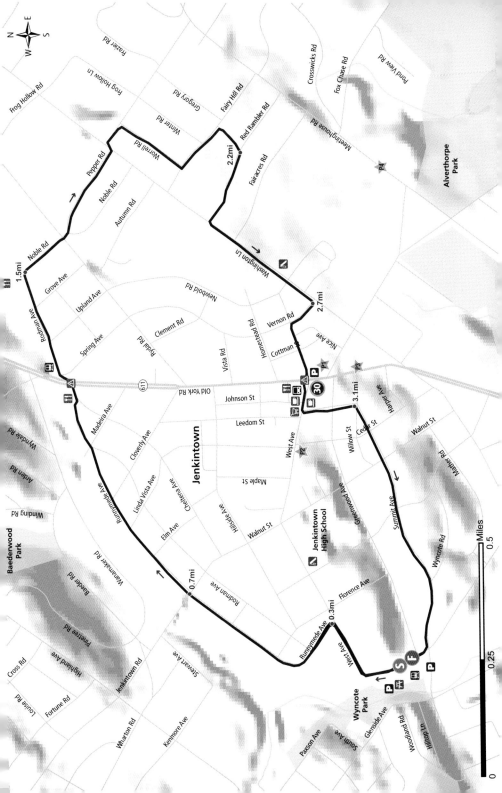

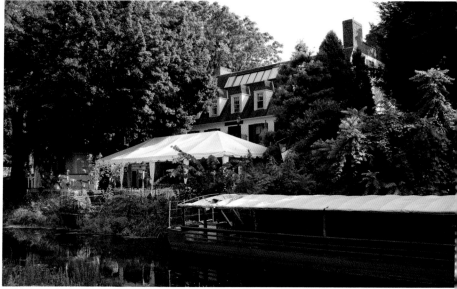

Dilly's Corner by the Center Bridge.

At a Glance

Distance 14.0 miles   **Total Elevation** 128 feet

Terrain

The trails run parallel to the Delaware River and are therefore generally flat. You'll ride through dirt, gravel, pebbles, and even some grass.

Traffic

The sections around New Hope and Lambertville are probably the busiest in terms of bike/ped traffic. You will hop on-road for a couple of blocks to cross the Delaware River.

How to Get There

Drive. I know, I'm sorry. There is metered street parking all over New Hope, and a $5 all day parking lot at the entrance to the towpath on Ferry Street.

Food and Drink

There are only a million excellent places to stop for a bite along this ride – there are options at the trail junctions in Lumberville, Stockton, Lambertville, and of course in New Hope. Zoubi's, just a block away from the start point on the corner of Mechanic and New streets, has awesome snacks and strong coffee.

Side Trip

Take a stroll through lovely New Hope! You'll be treated to some terrific people-watching on the main streets and in the shops and cafés sprinkled all over town.

Where to Bike Rating

About...

With 30 miles each in Pennsylvania and New Jersey, the canal trails run parallel alongside the Delaware River. There are five bridges that connect the trails, granting you the freedom to choose ride lengths between six and 60 miles (the Pennsylvania path runs from Uhlerstown to Morrisville and the New Jersey path from Frenchtown to Trenton). The ride log includes options for six and 14 mile loops, both of which begin in New Hope.

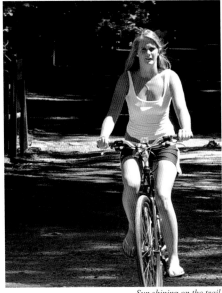

Sun shining on the trail.

Bucks & Montgomery Counties

The entrance to the towpath in New Hope is so easy to find that folks gave me a funny look when I asked for directions; it is situated underneath the tiny Ferry Street Bridge on the corner of Ferry and Stockton. The directions from here are easy – head north. When you tire, cross the Delaware, and head south in New Jersey.

The Pennsylvania side is known as the Delaware Canal State Park, and the New Jersey side is referred to as the Delaware and Raritan Canal State Park.

On the Pennsylvania side, you'll pedal along the geese laden Delaware Canal. From the 1830s to the 1930s, the canal was a busy passage for anthracite coal and lumber. Being here feels like a throwback to an earlier America – especially in the mornings when the path is empty. Duck as best you can under the bridges that crisscross the towpath, as some have surprisingly low clearances! And, try to watch out for poison ivy in the summer.

The path is quite narrow in the first section, and mostly covered with dirt and small pebbles. The Centre Bridge is your first option to reach New Jersey, bringing you back to New Hope in a short six mile loop. If you cross this bridge, you'll find yourself in quaint Stockton, N.J. There are plenty of places to stop for a rest or have a snack in Stockton before making a right to head back south on the trail.

Your next option to cross into New Jersey is the pedestrian bridge, known to some as the Raven Rock Bridge, in Lumberville. But remember, after the Centre Bridge, the gravel gets bigger! You will enjoy this 14 mile loop, if you have proper tires to handle the gravel.

The seven miles home on the New Jersey side (if you cross the Raven Rock) is fast and fun, again with smaller pebbles. When you reach Lambertville, the trail ends in a parking lot as new development creeps up to the very edge of the park. Stay straight until you see the bridge that takes you back over the river and into New Hope. You'll have a few blocks of on-road riding here to get back to the start, but if uncomfortable, there's no shame in walking your bikes right to the doorstep of Zoubi's!

Ride Log

0.0 Start out on the New Hope Towpath just behind Mechanic St and Stockton Ave. There's really only one way to go here – so head north!

0.8 The path narrows as you ride under one of many bridges to come. Enjoy your long stay on the towpath.

3.1 Arrive at Dilly's Corner and the Centre Bridge Inn, again to the left of the canal. If you only want to ride six miles today, then cross the Delaware using the Centre Bridge (just ahead) to pick up the Delaware and Raritan Canal State Park trail in New Jersey. From here, follow directions at mile 10.3. If you want to ride on, keep straight on the towpath.

3.2 After Center Bridge, the path is much wider and far quieter. It also changes from dirt to gravel.

6.3 You'll see the Raven Rock pedestrian bridge across the river, and voila! Lumberville!

6.4 Pedal just a hair beyond the pedestrian bridge and make a hairpin left onto River Rd to track back to the entrance. You'll see the Lumberville General Store ahead. Take the bridge over the river to New Jersey.

6.7 Continue straight after the bridge. You'll pass by the Bulls Island State Park parking area.

6.9 Make a right to pick up the Delaware and Raritan Canal State Park path and head back south. Noisy but beautiful birds are in residence here during the summer, keeping you company as you pedal along this straightaway for quite a bit.

10.3 Stockton junction. There's a small deli on the corner to grab a snack or cold drink. Ready to go? Keep heading south (if you've just come off the Centre Bridge, south is to the right).

12.5 The path turns into a humorously overgrown dirt and grass trail.

13.4 Exit the path and ride through the parking lot, then keep straight on the street all the way to Bridge St in Lambertville.

13.6 Make a right to cross the bridge (there's a walkway for bikes).

14.0 Left on Main St, and then another right on Ferry St to take you back to the start point. Or, bike one block farther to visit the dessert case at Zoubi's on Mechanic St!

P1 Bucks County Playhouse
70 South Main Street, New Hope
P2 Bulls Island State Park
P3 Holcombe-Jimison Farmstead Museum
1605 Daniel Bray Hwy, Lambertville

B1 New Hope Cyclery
404 Lower York Rd, New Hope, PA
BR1 Pure Energy Cycling and Java House
99 South Main St, Lambertville, NJ

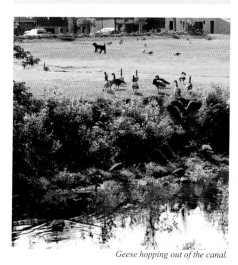

Geese hopping out of the canal.

The Pennsylvania & New Jersey Canal Loop Trails

Altitude ft

200
100
0

0   2   4   6   8   10   12   14.0

Distance miles

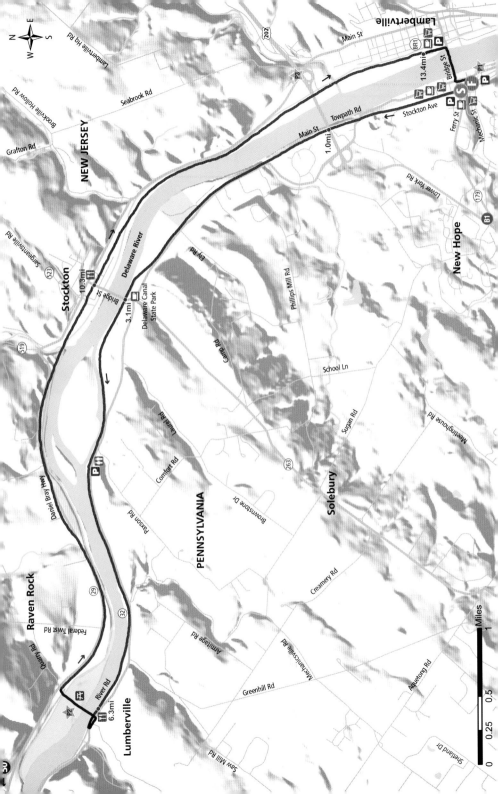

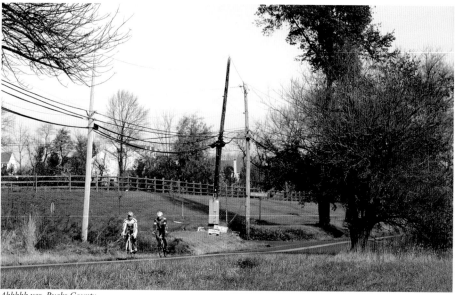

Ahhhhh yes, Bucks County.

At a Glance

Distance 19.6 miles   **Total Elevation** 597 feet

Terrain

Whew! This is one hilly ride. Enjoy! You'll be primarily on road, save for a couple of miles through Peace Valley Park. There are lots of good shoulders around here – you'll have plenty of room to crank up your speed and race the cars.

Traffic

While a few of these streets are very quiet, most will have traffic. Some streets, including Court Street and Main Street, have quite a bit of traffic. Stay cool!

How to Get There

Take the Septa Doylestown line to, you guessed it, Doylestown! The train ride is about an hour from Center City Philadelphia. There is also ample parking at the station.

Food and Drink

The bustling center of Doylestown has a number of excellent restaurants and quick places to stop for something to eat. Once on the road though, options are fewer and farther between. Be sure to pack a snack for extra energy on those hills.

Side Trip

Visit the James A. Michener Art Museum, which has permanent collections of Bucks County art as well as unique rotating exhibits. You can learn about Bucks County writers, composers, artists, actors and designers in their massive database. For more information, visit michenermuseum.org.

Where to Bike Rating

About...

Here is another chance to try Septa's Bike and Ride program – the ride log for this loop starts at the Doylestown train station. Check out this ride if you've never been up this way; Doylestown and the surrounding area of Bucks County is simply stunning. Thanks to George and Hugh Clark, and to Todd Baylson, for suggesting this ride, originally created as part of a fundraiser named "Bike for Barak" in 2008.

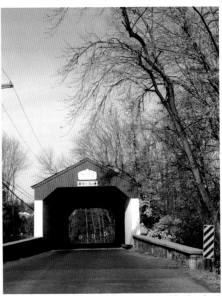

One of the many covered bridges here.

Bucks & Montgomery Counties

Your train ride to Doylestown will take about an hour from Center City. After you hop off, grab a snack at the station café, stretch out your legs and get ready! This is an awesome 20 mile loop.

Doylestown came to be in 1745, when William Doyle opened a watering hold on what is now the corner of Main Street and East State Street. Today, the town offers up a historic vibe with its old brick buildings, tree lined streets, and quaint shops and cafés. Don't miss County Theater – a restored blue and yellow Art Deco movie theater on East State Street.

The log begins in the center of Doylestown. On your way out of town you'll ride through residential streets lined with historic brick buildings. West Court Street and Almshouse Road will be slightly busier than others, but soon you'll be riding along the kind of quiet, gorgeous roads that cyclists dream of. Plus you get to ride through the red covered bridge on Old Iron Hill Road.

One highlight of this trip is Peace Valley Park (see Kids' ride 16 for more information about the area). You'll reach the entrance around mile five, and enjoy a long loop around Lake Galena before popping back out on the road and cycling through some of the more rural areas of Bucks County.

The next few miles of the ride has a lot of ups and downs – a few steep climbs, and some long rolling hills. You'll pedal past horses, farmland, and wide open spaces that will make you feel like you could turn those wheels for days and days!

As you make your way back to the center of Doylestown, you may find some of the roads aren't as well marked as is preferable. I did take a few wrong turns – East Court Street and North Church Street were particularly confusing – but folks were super gracious about helping me on my way. If you hit Main Street, you are in the clear (it might not be as desirable riding as some of the other side streets, due to its traffic, but the train station is nearby). Once you find Bridge Street, you'll be back at the station, and no doubt ready for another snack and a stretch!

Ride Log

0.0 Coming out of the parking lot, make a left on Clinton St.

0.1 Left on Oakland Ave.

0.4 Right on Lafayette St.

0.5 Left on W Court St. This is a busier road! It becomes Lower State Rd.

2.3 Lower State Rd becomes Almshouse Rd.

4.0 Right on the very small Sioux Rd.

4.1 Quick left on Keeley Ave. This becomes Old Iron Hill Rd. Pedal through the beautiful Pine Run covered bridge.

5.3 Left on Creek Rd, which runs along the edge of Peace Valley Park.

5.9 Right on Callowhill Rd.

6.4 Right on New Galena Rd. Bike through Peace Valley Park.

8.2 Exit Peace Valley, make a right to stay on New Galena Rd.

10.0 Right at the T-intersection to pick up W Swamp Rd.

10.1 Quick Left on Curly Hill Rd.

11.8 Cross Old York Rd. Use caution.

12.0 Cross Old Easton Rd, remain on Curly Hill Rd.

12.8 Right on Valley Park Rd.

14.2 Right on Point Pleasant Pike.

15.4 Left on Old Easton Rd.

17.5 Left at the light on W Swamp Rd.

17.7 Right on North St.

18.1 Left on East St.

18.5 Right on E Court St.

18.8 Left on N Church St.

19.0 Right on E State St.

19.3 Left on S Main St. You'll be riding through the center of Dolyestown here.

19.5 Right on Bridge St.

19.6 Arrive at the Doylestown train station.

 P1 James A Michener Art Museum, 138 South Pine St, Doylestown
P2 Peace Valley Nature Center, 170 North Chapman Rd, Doylestown
P3 County Theater, 20 East State St, Doylestown
P4 Pine Run covered bridge

 B1 Cycle Sports of Doylestown, 641 North Main St, Doylestown
B2 High Road Cycles of Doylestown, 73 Old Dublin Pike #4, Doylestown

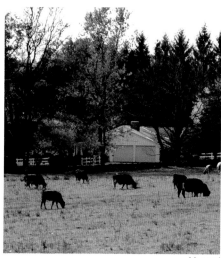

Mooooo!

The Doylestown "Bike for Barak" Ride

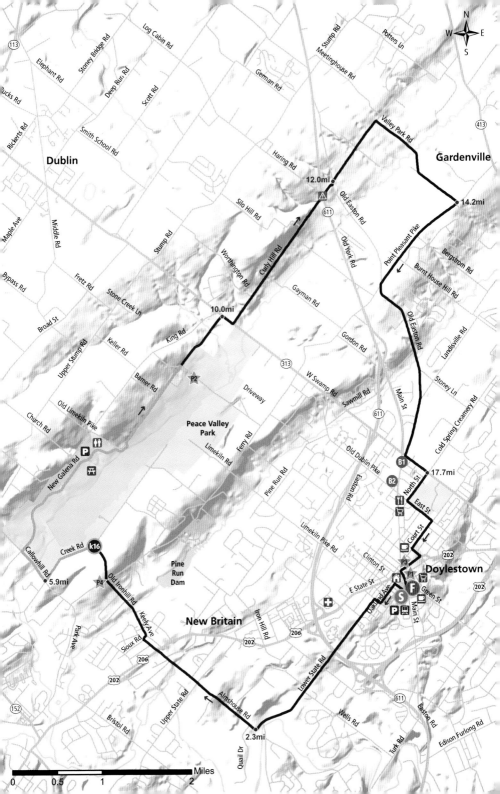

All Those Western 'Burbs

If you are looking for long rural and suburban rides, then this is the section for you. Covering terrain in Delaware, Chester, and Lancaster counties, these rides will take you from town to country in a few miles, and leave you wondering how all this rugged beauty could possibly exist so close to the city.

A really big thanks goes out to Viktor Ohnjec from the West Chester Cycling Club, and to Thomas Madle from the Bicycle Club of Philadelphia for suggesting routes. They've graciously condensed their years of pedaling into a few excellent loops for you.

Additionally, the PASA Bike Fresh Bike Local (Ride 40) is particularly scenic and should be of interest to local food enthusiasts and beer drinkers alike – the ride begins and ends at Victory Brewing and takes you through the hilly farmland of Lancaster County. Rides 37, 38, and 39 are similarly soul soothing as you make turn by turn in horse country.

You'll smile from ear to ear when you see another cyclist alongside you in an otherwise quiet, serene backdrop. They seem to pop up when you least expect it out here! Whichever route you choose for your inaugural ride, you'll definitely want to stop at some beautiful spot and take an extra five minutes to eat your peanut butter crackers.

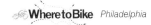

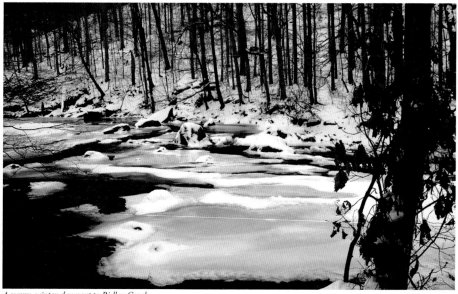

A sunny, winter day next to Ridley Creek.

At a Glance

Distance 4.2 miles   **Total Elevation** 410 feet

Terrain

Ridley Creek Park provides a multiuse, paved path that loops around the woods. One section of the path has a very steep downhill, and the remainder gets your heart pumping with a slow incline.

Traffic

This park is usually packed – I went in the dead of winter and was surprised to be in the company of many other cyclists, runners, and hikers.

How to Get There

Ridley Creek is located in Media, about 15 miles west of the city. Not a ton of public transit options to get here, so it might be best to pack up the car and drive on out. Lots 7, 11, 15, and 17 will give you access to the trail, as well as the lot at the park office (the address is 351 Gradyville Road in Newtown Square).

Food and Drink

This ride is a great excuse for a big, delicious picnic. Shady places to stop for a rest abound, in addition to 14 designated picnic areas with charcoal grills.

Side Trip

Check out the Tyler Arboretum, located adjacent to Ridley Creek State Park. The arboretum provides 650 acres of rare and ancient trees, and there is year 'round programming for the whole family.

Where to Bike Rating

About...

There is quite a bit to do in Ridley Creek State Park, including 12 miles of hiking trails through the woods, formal gardens near the entrance, summer fishing in Ridley Creek, and sledding and cross-country skiing when snow covers the ground. The paved multi-use trail along Sycamore Mills and Forge Road are very popular for biking, and it provides city-dwellers with a relatively close (only 16 miles from Center City!) option for a change of scenery.

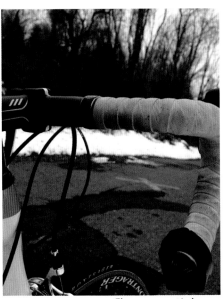

Gloves are a must in January.

There are plenty of places to begin your adventure, but a put-in near the park office is centrally located and easy to find. Park in the lower lot and look for the sign marking the trail. You'll have to walk your bike for just a bit on the hiking trail to reach the paved trail.

Once you arrive at the paved trail, you have a major decision to make. Do I turn right, or do I turn left? If you turn right, you'll have a slow steady climb for three and a half miles of your trip with a steep half mile downhill in the middle. If you choose left, you'll be coasting downhill for most of the ride but then be faced with a super steep incline. Your call! Of course, the log supposes you've made a right turn.

The path can be narrow at times and it is well traveled, so be sure to call out when passing. The area near the steep hill is a little wider, so even though it seems like a good idea to burn it, there are strict speed limits for bicycles on the downhill.

The highlight of the loop is the section along the beautiful Ridley Creek. The photos are from a cold winter day, but I imagine this place to be green and lush in the summertime. It's stocked in season with trout, and fishing is very popular.

After the river, a few more curves and steady incline will bring you back to the put-in.

A section of the park is on the National Register and has been designated the "Ridley Creek State Park Historic District" for its 18th century structures. The Colonial Pennsylvania Plantation, a 'living history' center showcasing one of the oldest working farms in Pennsylvania, is a fun place to visit. Guests are welcome April – November.

If you'd like to be more involved, The Friends of Ridley Creek State Park hosts volunteer days, trail maintenance mornings, tours and annual social events.

All Those Western 'Burbs

Ride Log

 P1 Hunting Hill Mansion and Garden
P2 Historic area, Sycamore Mills
P3 Fishing Platforms

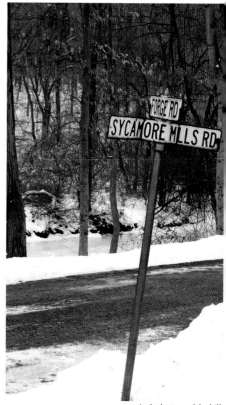

0.0 Hop on the trail by the put-in near the park office mansion.

0.1 Make a right if you wish to take the loop uphill, or a left if you wish to take it downhill. The log follows the path if you were to take a right.

0.7 There is a small fork here – follow the trail to the left. If you take the straight path to the right, you'll end up at the Rt 352 exit – nope you don't want to ride there! For the next little bit, the path is narrow and curves quite a lot.

1.5 Path straightens out as you follow E Forge Rd.

2.2 Welcome to an awesome downhill! It's very easy to get your speed up here, so be sure to stay in control.

2.7 Take the switchback at the bottom of the hill. The sign will direct you towards Sycamore Mills Rd. Now you'll begin to follow the Ridley Creek.

3.4 The path veers away from the river as you climb.

4.2 Back to the put-in.

At the bottom of the hill.

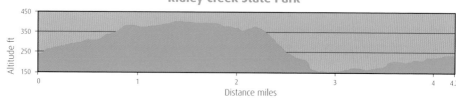

Ridley Creek State Park

Altitude ft

Distance miles

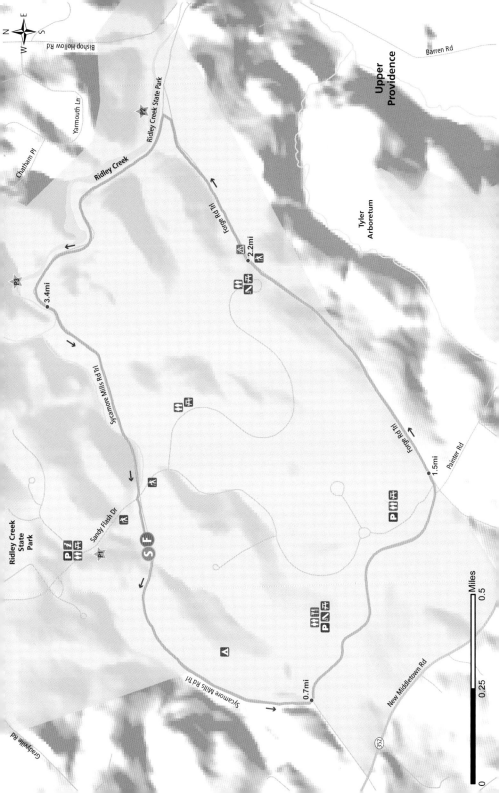

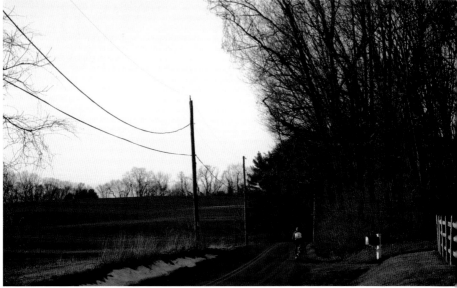

A fellow December rider.

At a Glance

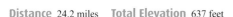

Distance 24.2 miles   **Total Elevation** 637 feet

Terrain

Grab some extra water – this ride takes you through a pretty hilly area of West Chester. Not too many extreme spikes, but definitely a lot of ups and downs and long, rolling hills.

Traffic

As with many suburban rides, these roads will not have as much traffic as those in the city, but I sometimes find the cars to be way bigger and moving a heck of a lot faster.

How to Get There

East Goshen Park is located off Paoli Pike in West Chester, and it has a big parking lot. Driving is probably your best bet, though Regional Rail will take you to the Malvern train station, located at mile 19.6 in the log.

Food and Drink

There are a couple of small cafés in Malvern, including Marie's coffee shop and Catalina's. You'll also pass a convenience store or gas station every few miles if you find yourself low on water or peanut butter crackers.

Side Trip

Check out Pete's Produce, a big 'ol farmstand near Cheyney University. Pete's sells tons of local fruits and vegetables in season, plus yummy baked goods for the road.

Links to 39

Where to Bike Rating

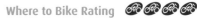

About...

This is a lovely ride around West Chester that overlaps with some of Ride 39; Okehocking Hills. You will start in East Goshen Park making your way out of the suburbs and on towards the rolling hills of Westtown. On the way home, the ride will bring you through the heart of Malvern, a little town with a few lunch options. This loop is a great introduction to the area if you've never cycled here before.

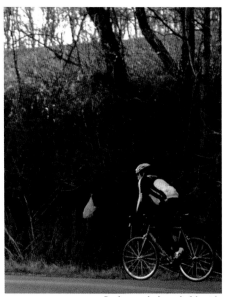

Dusk towards the end of the ride.

And now, a brief thank you to Mr. Viktor Ohnjec, member of the West Chester Cycling club and a master of Chester County rides. Dear Viktor: Thank you for introducing me to your neck of the woods. Your rides (36, 37, and 38) are tops, and I hope folks will venture out to beautiful West Chester for its idyllic scenery and fun change of pace.

This ride begins at East Goshen Park, a big open space with a long walking loop and a ton of adorable dogs. You'll ride out through the suburbs into a more rural area of West Chester. There are some funky streets here – not every stretch will be as perfectly paved as you might like – but for the most part you'll find these to be excellent roads for cycling. You're likely to especially enjoy Creek , Westtown , and Manley roads.

There are two loops to this ride; one above West Chester Pike and one below. The first loop takes you through East Goshen and Malvern. The second loop winds through Westtown and Cheney. They are connected by Manley and Dutton Hill Road, and you'll have to cross both Street Road and West Chester Pike to get to the second loop – be sure to use caution at these busy intersections.

Viktor refers to the route as "A Good Kids 24 Mile Loop." He must be talking about some hearty kids! I assume he refers to the route as such because of the safety of the roads and their general low traffic, as opposed to the terrain. Don't be embarrassed if you start sucking wind on some of the hills, especially around mile 11 and mile 18.

If you're looking for a shorter ride, then you can follow the first loop across Line Road for a 12 mile trek that will take you through Malvern. This might be a nice option for a short afternoon spin if you are taking the train from Center City – the ride passes the Malvern train station at mile 20.

Ride Log

0.0 Start at East Goshen Park, follow TWP Park across Paoli Pike.

0.1 Straight on Hibberd Ln. This is a very suburban area.

0.7 Continue on Clock Tower Dr.

1.2 Right on Peach Tree Dr at the T-intersection.

1.5 Left on Towne Dr.

2.1 Right on Line/Township Line.

2.7 Right on Dutton Mill Rd.

3.1 Right on Manley Rd.

4.6 Left on Ponds Edge Rd.

5.0 Follow the curve in the road.

5.4 Left on Walnut Hill Rd.

6.6 Right on Street Rd, but just for a minute. Be careful here!

6.8 Left on Cheyney Rd.

7.5 Right on Creek Rd.

7.8 Continue on Westtown Rd for a bit here.

10.43 Right on Westtown Way.

11.1 Hard right on Walnut Hill Rd.

11.2 Quick left on Manley Rd. Stay on Manley for close to two miles.

13.2 Left on Dutton Mill Rd.

13.9 Bear left on Line/Township Line.

14.4 Right on Chowning Dr.

14.8 Left on Dutton Mill Rd.

15.5 Left on Sugartown Rd.

15.5 Quick right on Spring Rd. Pedal here for two miles; it will become Jaffrey Rd.

17.6 Left on Grubb Rd – another two mile stretch.

19.6 Left on East King Rd. You'll ride through downtown Malvern – and pass a Septa station if pooped out.

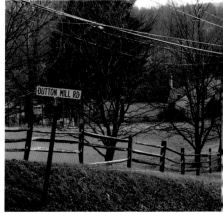
Good 'ol Dutton Mill Road.

P1 East Goshen Park
P2 Cheyney University
P3 Pete's Produce,
  1225 East Street Rd, West Chester

B1 Performance Bicycle Shop,
  1740 E Lancaster Ave, Paoli
B2 West Chester Bicycle Center,
  1342 West Chester Pike #B, West Chester

20.3 Left on Warren Ave (Septa on right).

20.4 Right on Monument Ave. Marie's café is on the corner.

21.9 Continue on Willow Pond Rd.

22.1 Continue on Line/Township Line.

22.9 Right on Warrior Rd.

23.2 Left on Taylor Ave.

23.7 Right on Paoli Pike.

24.2 Right into East Goshen Park – Done!

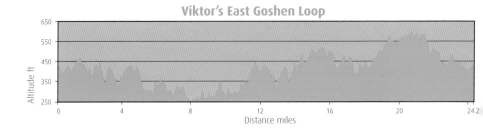

Viktor's East Goshen Loop

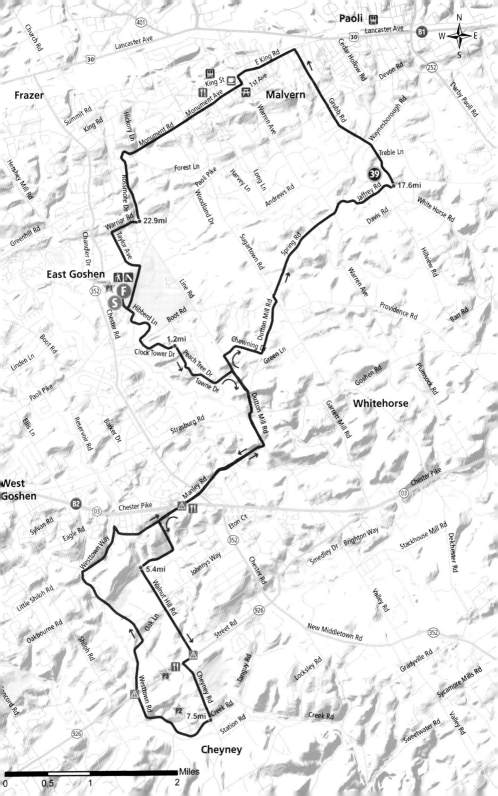

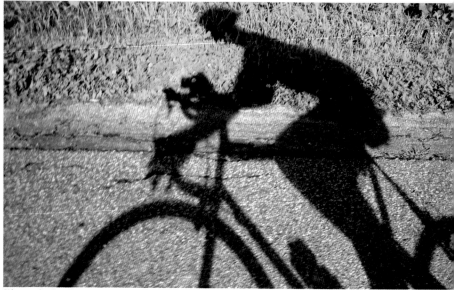

Viktor on his bicycle.

At a Glance

Rural Ride

Distance 14.4 miles   **Total Elevation** 521 feet

Terrain

The single scoop is mostly rolling hills with one good ascent around mile 12. The ride is all on-road.

Traffic

Traffic will be a bit heavier as you ride through the center of West Chester, but much quieter once you leave town. Cars move pretty fast on these roads though – be sure to have a lot of reflective gear at the ready.

How to Get There

If driving, head west on Route 202 from Philadelphia – the Single Scoop and Double Scoop have some of the furthest start points from the city. Buses 92, 104, and 306 will bring you to West Chester.

Food and Drink

Most of the food and drink options for this ride are in downtown West Chester, though there are one or two outposts along the way. Be sure to save some room fo ice cream at West Chester Scoops!

Side Trip

Check out The Note in West Chester. It's a small mu sic and comedy venue that occasionally has some de cent acts come through, including concerts hosted by WXPN.

Links to 38

Where to Bike Rating

About...

The shorter of the two, the West Chester Single Scoop starts in downtown West Chester and brings you through some of the surrounding suburbs. The roads are beautiful, and once you leave West Chester the traffic is generally mild. You are also certain to see plenty of other cyclists along the way. This is the second of Viktor's rides, so be sure to check out 36 and 38 if you like his style.

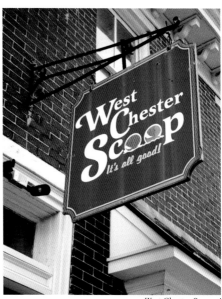

West Chester Scoops!

You'll start off on Darlington Street by West Chester Scoops and take Gay and New streets out of the center of town. There are plenty of cyclists in this area, but the streets are narrow and not all of the stops are four-way (many a time has a driver with the right of way honked at me in West Chester!).

Take your time leaving the center of town. Soon enough you'll find yourself on the residential roads of Sconnelltown, Barnhill, and St. Finnegan. These roads are very quiet, and they sneak up on you quickly. Be sure to keep an eye out for the next turn as you ride through this neighborhood.

The ride picks up speed on Creek Road, becoming more scenic as well. Creek Road is an excellent road for bicycles, you're sure to enjoy it!

Next comes the intersection around Bridge Road/ Route 842, which can be confusing the first time. Be sure to follow the signs and riding log closely, and you'll be on your way towards Wawaset.

You'll continue along these beautiful, rural roads for the next few miles. The terrain will be quite varied here. Expansive landscapes with red barns, horses and green pastures provide an idyllic picture postcard backdrop. The two miles on Lucky Hill Road is very

enjoyable, and you'll be able to relax for a bit on your bike without having to worry about the next turn coming your way!

After Miner, the turn for Price Street sneaks up. Take note: It's a very hard right, and one that I missed a couple of times! The sign is small. If you miss Price, you'll cross Bradford Avenue. Price will bring you back into West Chester (again, use caution while heading into town). You'll arrive back at WC Scoops on Darlington Road ready for a scoop!

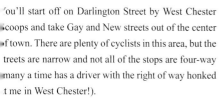

All Those Western 'Burbs

Ride Log

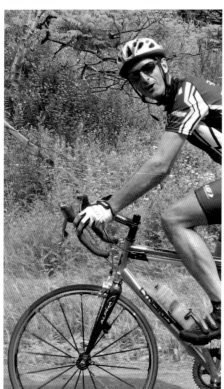

Viktor wants an entire sundae.

0.0 Start at West Chester Scoops, Gay St is just ahead
0.1 Left on Gay St.
0.2 Left on New St.
0.8 Right on Miner St.
1.0 Left on Sconnelltown Rd.
2.0 Left on Birmingham Rd.
2.2 Right on Marlin Dr.
2.8 Left on Barn Hill Rd.
3.0 Left on Muirfield Dr.
3.2 Right on St. Finegan Dr.
3.7 Right on S Creek Rd.
4.3 Left on Rt 842 (Bridge Rd).
4.7 Left on N Wawaset Rd.
6.1 Left on Camp Linden Rd.
6.7 Left on Northbrook Rd.
7.0 Right on Broad Run Rd.
8.0 Right on Clayton Rd.
9.1 Straight on Strasburg Rd.
9.6 Right on Lucky Hill Rd.
11.8 Left on Allerton Rd, then straight on Miner St (Rte 842).
13.3 Right on Price St.
14.0 Left on Darlington Rd.
14.4 Back at WC Scoops!

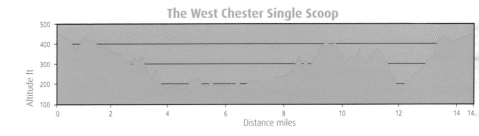

The West Chester Single Scoop

Altitude ft

Distance miles

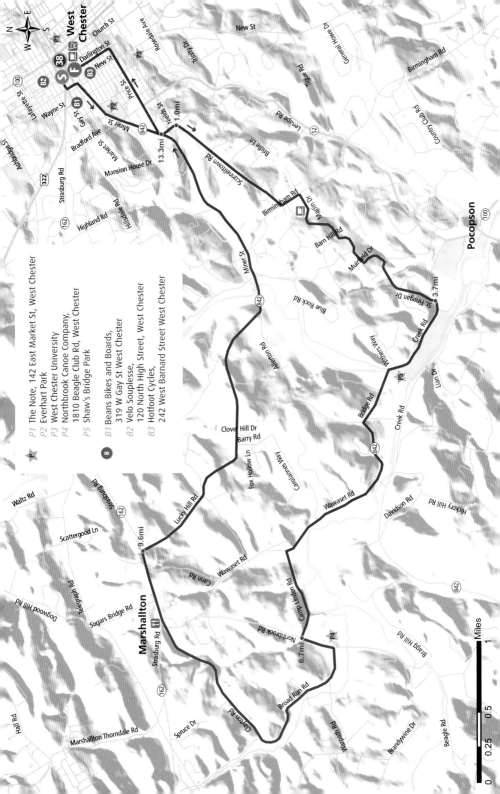

West Chester

P1 The Note, 142 East Market St, West Chester
P2 Everhart Park
P3 West Chester University
P4 Northbrook Canoe Company, 1810 Beagle Club Rd, West Chester
P5 Shaw's Bridge Park

B1 Beans Bikes and Boards, 319 W Gay St West Chester
B2 Velo Souplesse, 120 North High Street, West Chester
B3 Hotfoot Cycles, 242 West Barnard Street West Chester

Pocopson

Marshallton

Miles
0   0.25   0.5   1

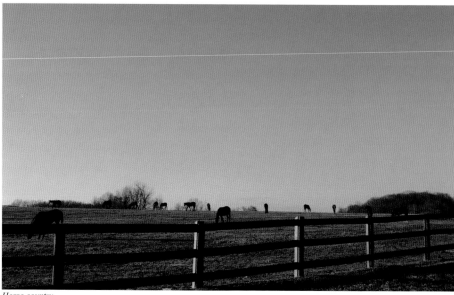

Horse country.

At a Glance

Distance 22.9 miles   **Total Elevation** 522 feet

Terrain

You'll bike on-road through hilly Chester County for the entirety of this trek. There are a couple steep spikes and lots of fast and furious downhills.

Traffic

There is steady traffic as you enter and exit the center of West Chester, but as you pedal farther away from West Chester Scoops, you'll enjoy roads with far fewer cars. Of course, as with the other rural rides, cars tend to move fast out here!

How to Get There

The Single Scoop and Double Scoop have some of the furthest start points from the city. Take Route 202 West towards West Chester. There is street parking all around West Chester Scoops, and Septa buses 92, 104, and 306 will bring you to the area.

Food and Drink

Downtown West Chester will be your best bet. It might be a good idea to grab a snack for the route! There are a few stops along the way, but for the most part, you'll be happy to have that soft pretzel in your bag.

Side Trip

You'll pass the Northbrook Canoe Company on Beagle Road – nothing could be finer than a bike ride with a tubing or kayaking trip down the Brandywine in between?

Links to ③⑦

Where to Bike Rating

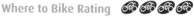

About...

The West Chester Double Scoop is one of the most scenic rides in the guide, and one of the hilliest as well. You are in for an ultra-satisfying 23 mile loop – excellent roads, a stunning backdrop, even the air smells differently out here! This is Viktor's third ride to make it into Where to Bike: Philadelphia – if you like his style, check out rides 36 and 37. Thanks again, V!

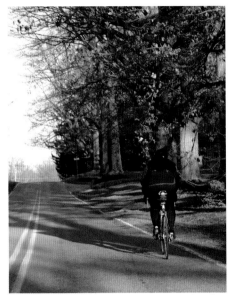

Low traffic roads makes for heavenly cycling.

Oh you long, luxurious rides of Chester County; Hilly, horsey, and green, you make us city dwellers want to move to the country forever! Or at least, hoof it out here for an awesome afternoon ride.

You'll start out at West Chester Scoops, as in Ride 37, and pedal straight out of West Chester. Again, there are some weird intersections that feel like they should be four way stops, but are not. Use caution as you make your way out of town.

The roads open up as soon as you hit North Creek Road, which also happens to be PA Bicycle Route L. There are considerable hills at mile 1, 3.4, and mile 5, so throw your low gear and put your head down; you'll enjoy the downhills that follow.

The roads are quiet and scenic through Maple Ridge, Lenape, and Indian Hannah. Some could use a good pave, and some are a touch narrower than I might prefer, but on the whole these are near perfect cycling roads, and they will make you extraordinarily jealous of the West Chester Cycling Club (of which Viktor is a member).

The Northbrook Canoe Company is situated on a corner that you will simply love around mile 15. I took this ride in the fall but this whole area gives you wafts of summer and warm weather. There's a food shack here that's open on weekends and holidays, if you need a quick snack.

Heading back into West Chester, you'll travel along PA Bicycle Route L again, and then slowly watch the rural roads change to residential. After Finegan Drive, you'll be in a development – not much traffic but a lot of fast turns before you hit Sconneltown Road. The turn onto Price is quick, so be sure to watch for it, especially if you're tired and ready for ice cream.

Ride Log

0.0 Start at West Chester Scoops, head towards Gay St.

0.1 Left on Gay St.

0.4 Right on Everhart Ave.

0.5 Left on W Chestnut St. Keep straight – this turns into Hillsdale Rd, pedal on Hillsdale for the next 1.5 miles.

2.1 Left onto Creek Rd.

2.8 Right on Allerton Rd.

4.3 Bear right onto Rt 842.

4.8 Left on S Wawaset Rd (if you only care to ride 10 miles, head straight for Bridge St and pick up the directions at mile 17.5 below).

5.8 Right on Locust Grove Rd.

7.0 Left on Corrine Rd, then a very quick right back onto Locust Grove.

7.6 Right on Lenape-Unionville Rd. Pedal on this road for close to 2.5 miles.

10.0 Right on Doe Run Rd.

11.4 Right back onto Wawaset/Rte 842.

14.2 Left onto Northbrook Rd.

16.0 Right on Camp Linden Rd.

16.6 Hello Wawaset! Make a right back onto N Wawaset Rd.

17.5 Bear left onto Rt 842; follow S Bridge Rd signs.

18.4 Right on S Creek Rd (after Bridge Rd). You'll see signs for "Bicycle Route L".

19.0 Left on St. Finegan Dr – you'll be heading back towards town now. The next few turns are pretty fast as you wave through quiet residential streets.

19.5 Left onto Muirfield Dr.

19.8 Right on Saint Anne Way.

19.9 Right onto Barn Hill Rd.

20.0 Right onto Marlin Dr.

20.5 Left on Birmingham Rd.

20.7 Left onto Sconneltown Rd.

21.8 Right onto Miner St/Rt 842.

21.8 Make a very fast right onto Price St.

22.5 Left onto Darlington, bike through the center of West Chester and…

22.9 Time for ice cream!

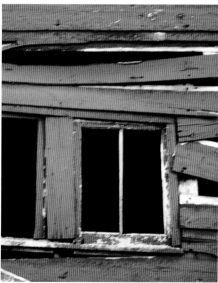

One of the many barns you'll pass along the way.

The West Chester Double Scoop

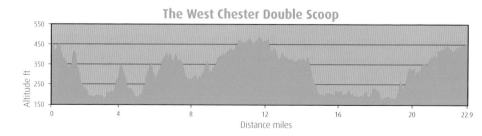

Altitude ft

Distance miles

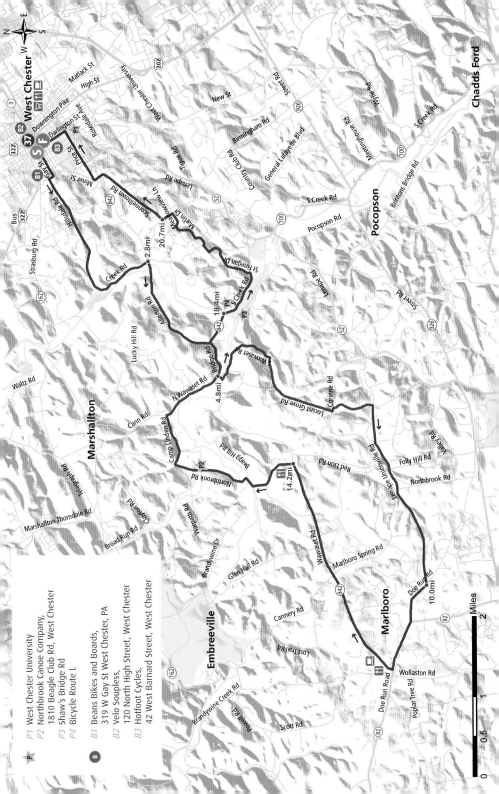

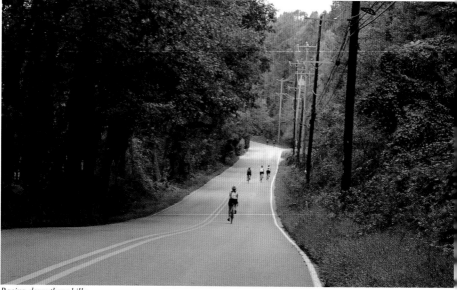

Racing down those hills.

At a Glance

Distance 32.0 miles   **Total Elevation** 571 feet

Terrain

Welcome to the hilliest ride in Where to Bike: Philadelphia! This one's beaut; all on road and one up and down after another.

Traffic

Traffic out here is fairly light, though you'll have to deal with a couple of big intersections (especially around Route 3 and 252).

How to Get There

The ride log starts at Church of our Savior in Wayne, located at 651 N Wayne Avenue. There's a huge parking lot here, so driving is a good bet. The train is also an option – the Paoli/Thorndale Septa line will drop you a few blocks away at Wayne station.

Food and Drink

Wayne is full of places to have a bite before or after your trip, but stops along the route itself are few and far between.

Side Trip

You'll pass the Okehocking Preserve, on West Chester Pike, about half way through this ride. It is a 180 acre open-space reserve; the perfect place to stop to stretch your legs and have a summer picnic.

Links to 36

Where to Bike Rating

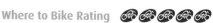

About...

This is a great ride to test your endurance and get your heart pumping. You'll cycle all over scenic Delaware County, and, in one of the most beautiful rides in the book, take in sweeping views of horse country at every turn. There are also options to shorten the ride if you just want a taste, or lengthen it if you're in love. This cue was suggested to me by long time ride leader for The Bicycle Club of Philadelphia, Tom Madle. Thanks, Tom!

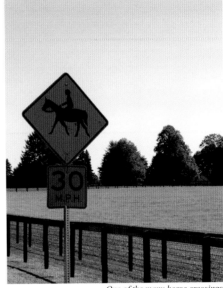

One of the many horse crossings.

The ride log begins in Wayne, very near to the downtown district along Lancaster Avenue. There are oodles of restaurants here to grab a bite before or after your trip, and lots of lovely shops too. If you take the train here, head up North Wayne Avenue from Lancaster Avenue to navigate your way to the starting point.

For the first few miles, you'll be riding along streets that are shady and curvy. A few have very tight shoulders, including Upper Gulph Road and West Valley Road. These roads will take you out to rather quiet residential streets like Bodine, Cypress, and Greene.

Around mile eight, you'll cross Lancaster Avenue and pass the Daylesford train station in the event of pooped-out-I-want-to-go-home syndrome. If you are still trucking, you'll soon pass Historic Waynesboro, and then, to your great pleasure, you will be in the heart of horse country. Warren Avenue, Providence Road, and Sugartown Road provide you with long stretches of rolling hills and drop dead gorgeous scenery.

If you wish to cut the ride short, simply make at left on Providence Road, rather than a right, at mile 12.7. Then pick up the ride log at 23.8 by making a left on Barr Road off of Providence. You'll eliminate the bottom 10 mile loop and still have a nice 22 mile ride on your hands.

If you're down for the full 32 miles, you'll pass the Okehocking Preserve at the corner of Delchester Road and Route 3/West Chester Pike. Be sure to use caution at this intersection! As you continue along Delchester, you'll ride adjacent to Ridley Creek State Park (Ride 35). Hop on over to add a few additional miles. Soon you'll begin to head back towards Wayne on very similar roads – hilly, shady, and with horses. Lovely.

Want to go even farther today? At mile 10.1 (Waynesboro and Grubb Road), you'll cross Ride 36: Viktor's East Goshen Loop, at its mile 18.1. Follow the log for Ride 36 all the way around again to 16.7 (Jaffrey / Spring roads and Warren Avenue) for an additional 23 biking miles. Make a right on Warren Avenue to pick up Ride 39 again, now at mile 11.5. You'll have a hilly 55 mile loop on your hands!

A final aside – Tom's other ride is just as slammin' as this one. Check out his excellent trek from Chestnut Hill to Bryn Athyn, Ride 30.

Ride Log

0.0 Start at the church and make a left on Radnor-Street Rd.

0.9 Right at Croton Rd.

1.1 Left on DeWhitt Rd (caution here).

1.2 Right on General Washington Rd.

1.4 Left at Pugh Rd.

3.4 Right on Valley Forge Rd, and a quick left on Devon Rd.

3.6 Right on Berwyn-Baptist Rd.

3.7 Right on Devonshire Rd.

4.2 Right on Contention Ln.

4.5 Left on Westwind.

5.3 Left on Cassatt Rd.

5.5 Right on Cloverly.

5.9 Right on Howelville at the T, and then the first left at Bodine Rd.

6.4 Left on Cypress.

6.5 Right on Green Rd.

7.1 Left at Irish Rd.

7.5 Right at Conestoga Rd, then an immediate right on Old Lancaster Rd.

8.1 Cross Lancaster Ave at the light to stay on Glenn Ave.

8.3 Right on Berwyn – Paoli Rd.

8.7 Left on Sugartown Rd, and a quick right on Waynesboro (first right).

9.0 Cross Rt 252/Darby-Paoli Rd.

10.1 Left on Grubbs Rd (links with Ride 36).

10.7 Right on Jaffrey Rd.

11.5 Left on Warren Ave.

12.7 Right on Providence Rd.

13.7 Left on Sugartown Rd at the T.

14.8 Left on Goshen Rd.

15.1 Right on Delchester Rd.

16.5 Cross Rt 3/ West Chester Pk.

17.1 Right on Stackhouse Mill Rd.

18.3 Right on Valley Rd at the T.

18.8 Right on Street Rd.

19.2 Cross West Chester Pike/Rt 3. You'll be on Garrett Mill Rd.

20.6 Right on Goshen Rd at the T.

20.7 Left on Sugartown Rd.

21.9 Right on Providence Rd.

22.9 Cross Warren Ave.

23.8 Left on Barr Rd.

24.5 Left on Grubbs Mill Rd, and a quick right onto Whitehorse Rd.

25.7 Left on Wayland.

26.5 Left on Rt 252/Darby-Paoli Pike.

27.1 Right on Beaumont Rd.

28.3 Right on Church Rd.

28.7 Left on Ladderback Rd.

29.2 Right on S Valley Forge Rd.

29.3 Left on Maplewood Rd.

29.5 Left on West Wayne Ave.

30.6 Right on Bloomingdale Ave.

30.8 Left on Runnymeade Ave.

31.0 Left on S Wayne Ave. Cross Rt 30, and Eagle Rd. Church is ¼ mile past Eagle Rd.

32.0 Church on the right.

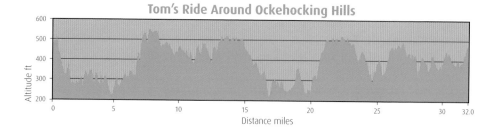

Tom's Ride Around Ockehocking Hills

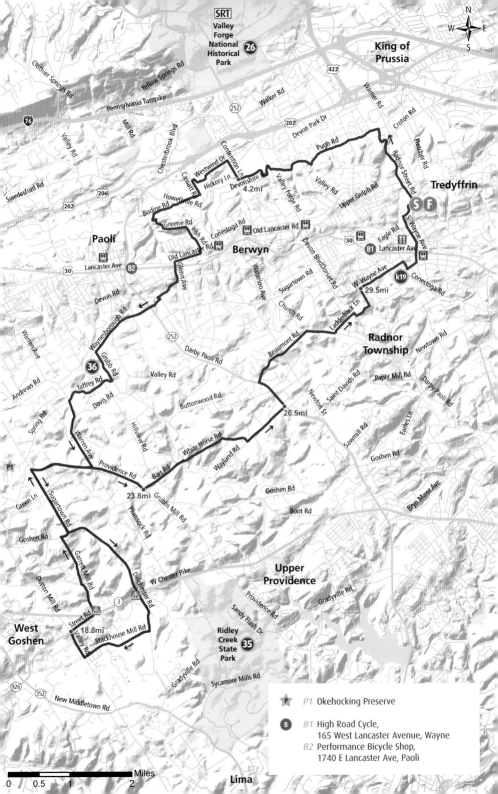

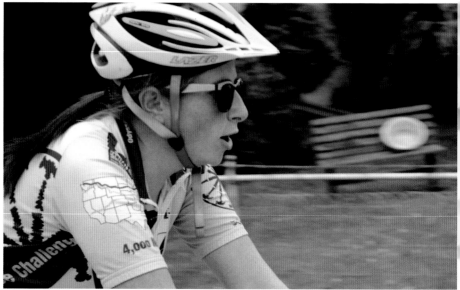

Biking fresh and local.

At a Glance

Distance 51.5 miles   **Total Elevation** 757 feet

Terrain

Dynamite hills and long roads with little traffic make up the lion's share of this unbelievable ride. It is all on road, save for the beginning on Struble Trail.

Traffic

The traffic is generally light, though you will encounter one or two roads with some fast cars.

How to Get There

The Downingtown Septa station is about a mile from Victory Brewing company, which is located at 420 Acorn Lane. If you drive, take Route 76 West. There is lots of parking at the brewery.

Food and Drink

Get real – go to Victory! You'll be starved by the time you return from your trek. Stops are few along the route itself, so be sure to pack a banana and 2 pb&j's.

Side Trip

Make a weekend out of it, and go camping in French Creek State Park! The park provides 7,730 acres of continuous forest (the largest block between NYC and DC!), with fishing, swimming, hiking, and wildlife, as well as cottages, yurts, and cabins that can be reserved for an overnight stay.

Links to   41

Where to Bike Rating

 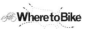

About...

Clocking in at 51.5 miles, the PASA Bike Fresh Bike Local is the longest ride in the book, and definitely a favorite. Chester County is cycling heaven – serene open spaces, long, well paved roads, graceful hills, crickets, trees, and adorable farm animals are everywhere. It's amazing to think this countryside is so close to Philadelphia. A bonus: PASA has marked most of the roads with little white arrows directing you where to turn.

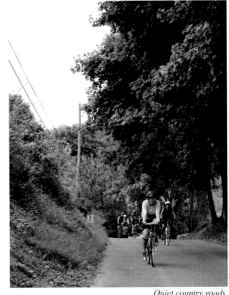

Quiet country roads.

A bit of background: PASA stands for the Pennsylvania Association for Sustainable Agriculture, a group that promotes local foods and family farms in our region. Bike Fresh Bike Local is their annual fundraiser. Marilyn Anthony, Southeast Regional Director of PASA, dreamed up the event along with Chef Royer Smith and Victory Brewing's Bill Covaleski. Her vision was a ride "that would engage the non-farming community and put them in touch with beautiful farmland and foods from those farms." The route was designed by the talented Eduardo Ruchelli, who was asked by PASA to include as much farm landscape as possible. Cyclists from all over the Mid-Atlantic region show up for the epic trek, which generally takes place in the fall.

But, now you can take this ride any day of the year! The cue is long, and all of the turns are very, very worth it. The log begins at Victory Brewing in Downingtown and picks up Struble Trail (Ride 41). You'll ride through Marsh Creek State Park as you head towards French Creek on some seriously perfect roads, including Bicycle Route L.

At mile 27.7, you'll hit French Creek State Park. It is a beautiful place for a rest, or a picnic, or a swim. If interested, make a right on Park Road to head towards French Creek. If you'd prefer to keep on cycling, then make a left on Park Road and pick up the log at mile 31. You'll continue along hills and farmland – with many scenic views along the way.

Soon you'll be on your way back to the brewery and ready for a cold drink. Take note: The last five miles along the shady, hilly Creek Road are a battle. Luckily, you'll be super close to Victory once you hit Pennsylvania Avenue.

A major thanks goes out to PASA, Marylin, Royer, Bill, and Eduardo for this gem. If you'd like more information about PASA, the next Bike Fresh Bike Local ride, or the sustainability and local foods movement in our region, check out www.pasafarming.org.

All Those Western 'Burbs

Ride Log

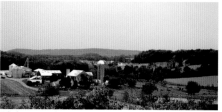

Oh the scenery!

0.0 Start at Victory Brewing. Make a left on Chestnut St.

0.1 Right on Lincoln Ave.

0.3 Right on Green St.

0.6 Right on Pennsylvania Ave.

0.7 Turn into parking lot and pick up Struble Trail.

3.7 Path ends. Make a left on Dorlan Mill Rd, and then a quick right on PA 282 (Creek Rd).

7.9 Right on Devereux Rd.

9.3 Make a right at the T onto Fairview Rd, then a quick left on Little Conestoga Rd.

11.4 Right on Adams Rd.

12.0 Left at the T to pick up Marsh Rd.

13.3 Right at the T onto Conestoga Rd.

13.4 Quick left onto Mansion Rd.

14.0 Bear right on James Mill Rd.

14.9 Left on Grove Rd.

15.1 Right on Dampman Rd.

15.9 Bear right on Warwick Furnace Rd.

19.0 Left at the T to pick up Coventryville Rd.

19.6 Left at Old Ridge Rd.

20.1 Right at the T onto PA23/Ridge Rd.

21.6 Right on St Peter's Rd.

21.8 Bear left to stay on St Peter's Rd.

23.1 Left on Harmonyville Rd.

23.5 Bear left to stay on Harmonyville (Keim Rd goes right).

24.5 Bear left again to stay on Harmonyville (Piersoll Rd goes right).

27.7 Make a right on Park Rd to head towards French Creek State Park (rest stop, picnic area). If not interested, make a left on Park Rd and pick up at mile 31.

29.3 Hit the lake! Turn around and hop back on Park Rd when you're finished with your rest.

31.0 Cross Harmonyville Rd.

32.3 Left on Ammon Rd.

33.0 Left at the T-intersection on PA82/Elverson Rd

35.7 Right on Bollinger Rd.

36.8 Bear left to stay on Bollinger.

38.0 Bear left at the Y to pick up Wyebrook Rd.

38.7 Left at Lewis Mills Rd.

38.9 Right on Reeder Rd.

39.1 Left on Killian Rd.

39.7 Left on Lippitt Rd, (becomes Indian Run Rd at PA82)

42.3 Right on Springton Rd.

43.9 Very sharp left at Highspire Rd (almost feels like a u-turn).

45.4 Right on PA 282 (Creek Rd). Ride along here for the next five miles.

50.7 Left on Pennsylvania Ave.

50.8 Right on Green St.

51.2 Left on Lincoln Ave.

51.4 Left on Chestnut St at the T-intersection, then a quick right on Acorn Ln.

51.5 Finish at Victory Brewing!

PASA's Bike Fresh Bike Local Tour

Please note profile for Ride 40 is depicted in 200ft vertical increments due to unusually high elevation.

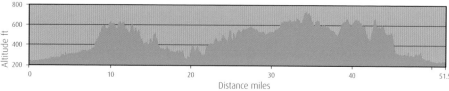

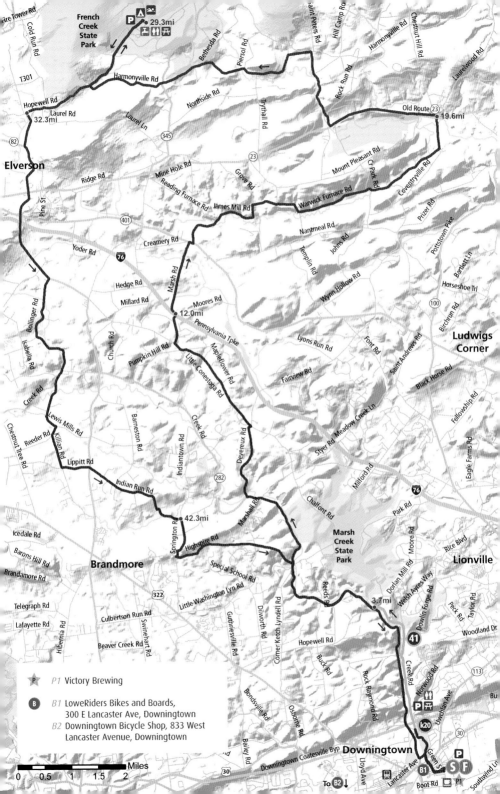

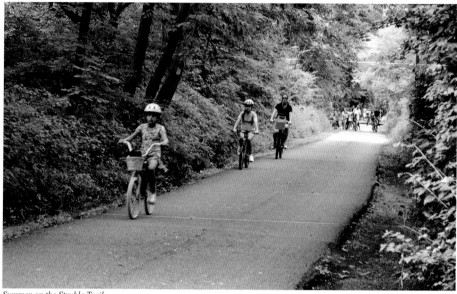

Summer on the Struble Trail.

At a Glance

Distance 8.4 miles   **Total Elevation** 424 feet

Terrain

The first portion of this bike path is flat, and the second has a steady incline. Struble Trail is much wider than the single lane Uwchlan, which weaves back and forth across Dowlin Forge and Pennypacker roads.

Traffic

These trails are very popular for running and cycling. Struble tends to have more little tykes than Uwchlan. There are a few blind turns (especially when traversing the road), so be a dear and stay to the right.

How to Get There

If driving from Philadelphia, head west to Downingtown. Parking is located just off the trail head on Norwood Road. The 204 Septa bus will drop you near the turnaround at Eagleview Corporate Park (you'll need to reverse the ride log if you take this bus).

Food and Drink

The hydration angels of The Downingtown Running Company place large water jugs along the trails on weekends in the summer. There are also a few cafés close to the turn around.

Side Trip

Marsh Creek State Park is very close by and provides lots of outdoor recreation options, including a 535 acre lake for fishing and boating, plenty of hiking trails, and a guarded swimming pool in the summer. It's a great place for ice skating and sledding in the winter too.

Links to

Where to Bike Rating

About...

The Struble and Uwchlan trails are heavily traveled, multi-use recreation paths in Chester County. A fun change of pace from city trails, they wind along the Brandywine and Shamona Creeks and pass by a few interesting stone ruins. Swinging from trees and jumping in the Brandywine are popular summer activities on Struble – what could be finer than a bike ride, a sandwich, and a dip in the creek on a warm afternoon?

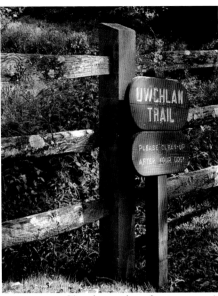

It's cool, no one knows how to pronouce it.

The trail starts just off Norwood Road in a parking lot so packed that you can call out your tire size and someone is guaranteed to have an extra tube. The Struble Trail is very nicely shaded and reasonably flat – it is a great path for a leisurely ride in the summer. There are plenty of well placed picnicking spots along the Brandywine, which runs parallel to the trail. If you take Struble to its end, you'll be very close to Marsh Creek State Park.

The turn to Uwchlan sneaks up – there is a small bridge, and you'll have to cross Dowlin Forge Road to find the entrance. You know you're heading in the correct direction when you pass the Grist Mill ruin to the right.

Uwchlan has a few funny turns and it is quite narrow. What begins as a shaded trail through the woods becomes a street-side path and ends in a development. The first time I took Uwchlan, I was convinced that I was heading in the wrong direction every few miles. But the arrows are well marked, when they do appear, so just stick to them as you cross back and forth over Shamona Creek and Dowlin Forge Road.

When you reach Dorian/S Milford Road, the path goes through a development and ends in the Eagleview complex (if you took the 204 bus, Eagleview will actually be your start point). There are a few cafés ahead if you're looking for a snack or a place to rest, including a coffee shop and bookstore with outdoor seating.

Most of Uwchlan is slightly uphill, so you'll be treated to a faster pace on the way home.

The Struble Trail was built atop the rail bed of the old Waynesburg Railroad in 1979, and was named for Robert G. Struble, former County Commissioner and Executive Director of the Brandywine Valley Association. These trails are part of a greater network that will eventually reach Glenmoor, Springton Manor Farm, and Honey Brook Borough – hooray! Currently, Struble and Uwchlan links to Spur Trail and Kardon Spur Trail.

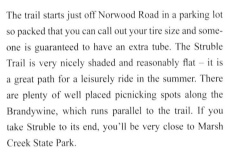

All Those Western 'Burbs

Ride Log

 P1 Kardon Park
P2 The Grist Mill

 B1 LoweRiders Bikes and Boards,
300 E Lancaster Ave, Downingtown

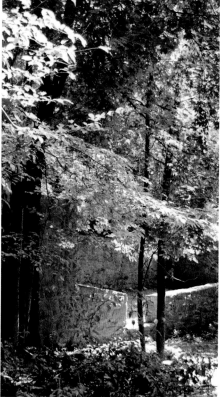

The old Grist Mill.

0.0 Start on the trail just off the very busy Norwood Ave parking lot. Follow the curves of the Brandywine Creek.

1.6 Make a right over the bridge to cross Dowlin Forge Rd and pick up Uwchlan Trail. It runs parallel to the street for a bit.

1.7 Beautiful remnants of the Grist Mill will be on your right. Head uphill for the next two miles – the Uwchlan Trail is much thinner than the Struble, and this portion follows the Shawmona Creek.

2.2 The path continues along Dowlin Forge Rd. Follow the signs as the path crosses the street back and forth.

3.0 Cross Kingston Ln and follow the path along Pennypacker Rd. Again, the trail will go back and forth across the street. Simply follow the cues.

3.5 Cross Dorian/S Milford Rd. You'll start to follow Rice Blvd. The teeny tiny path begins to resemble a sidewalk. There's a small shopping area ahead if you're looking for a snack or a coffee, otherwise, you may consider ending here and turning around.

4.0 Snacks to the right!

4.2 If you haven't yet started back, end here at Pennsylvania Dr (this is close to your start point if you took the bus).

4.9 Cross Dorian/S Milford Rd and follow Pennypacker Rd.

5.4 Cross Kingston Ln and follow the trail along Dowlin Forge Rd.

6.1 Follow the Shamona Creek home.

6.8 Cross Dowlin Forge Rd, and make a left to pick up the flat Struble Trail.

8.4 And home!

The Struble Trail & Uwchlan Trail

Altitude ft

600
500
400
300
200

0   2   4   6   8   8.4

Distance miles

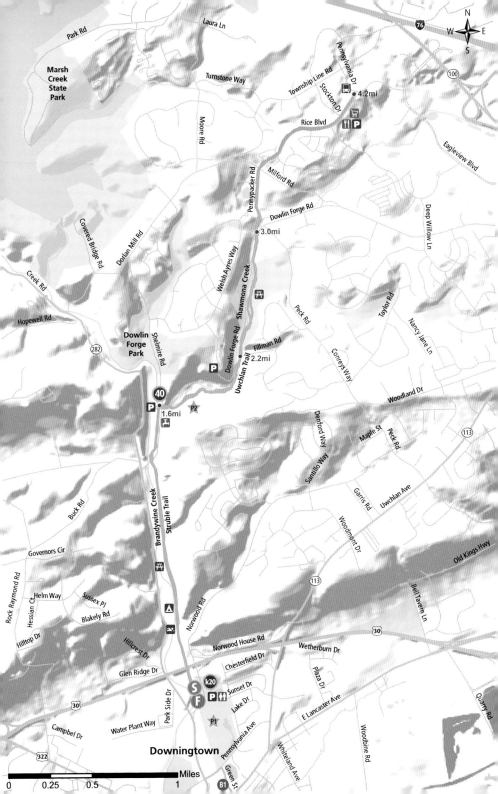

South Jersey

Most assuredly, the most wonderful bicycling surprises await you in South Jersey!

The rides in this section predominantly begin in Camden, Burlington, and Ocean counties. It's almost like road biking heaven out here; motorists give the impression that they are happy to offer cyclists the right of way. Wide bike shoulders and lanes pop up out of nowhere and go on for days. It's famously flat. And delicious snacks are specifically built in to almost every route.

Wait, snacks? Yes! The Old World Bakery has incredible coal fired pizza (Ride 46) and the Red Barn has pretty much the best pie in the world (Ride 45). The cyclists in South Jersey do it right – thank you to Joe Racite, David Wender and the other cyclists in the Outdoor Club of South Jersey and the Tri-County Cyclists and who offered suggestions for rides.

A couple of special rides in this section bring you all the way out to the shore. While the loops in Cape May (Ride 49) and Long Beach Island (Ride 48) may seem like a major travel commitment, they are well worth the trip. It doesn't get much better than taking your bike for a spin and jumping in the ocean on the same afternoon. These locations are good for both intense road riding and easy cruising along the water. Beat the crowds by visiting in the spring or fall, or have a blast alongside beachgoers in the summer.

Haven't been biking in South Jersey? Do it! You won't regret it, not at all!

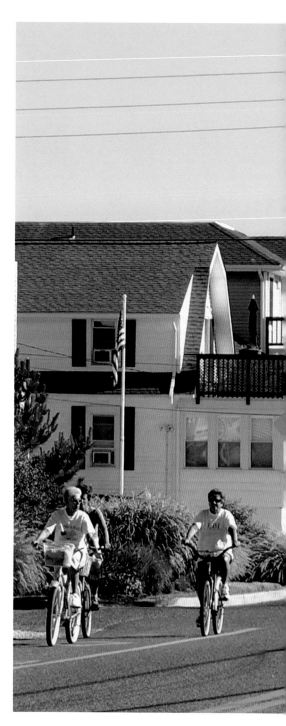

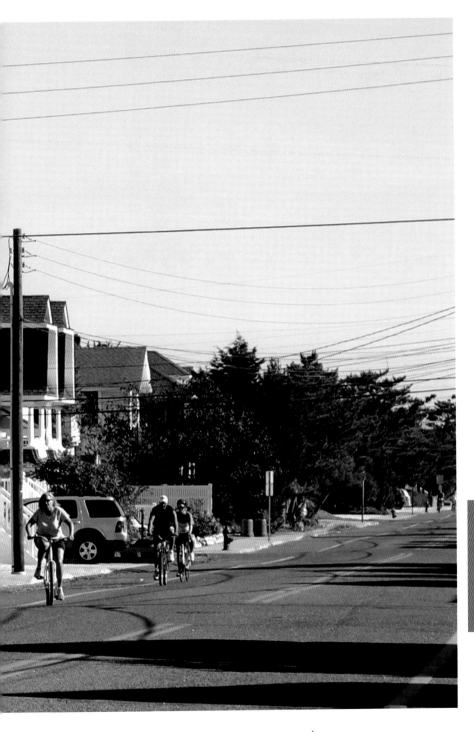

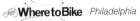

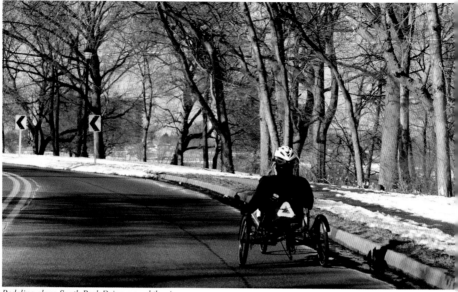

Pedaling along South Park Drive around the river.

At a Glance

Distance 3.8 miles   **Total Elevation** 27 feet

Terrain

This is one flat ride! Families will enjoy the paved path, while faster riders might prefer the wide roads that run alongside the path.

Traffic

There are always folks out enjoying Cooper River. The path sees its fair share of runners, walkers, cross-country skiers, strollers, and of course, cyclists. The roads adjacent to the path have slow, steady traffic, but drivers here seem very much accustomed to sharing the road.

How to Get There

The Ferry Avenue PATCO station is nearby on Colt Avenue, but you'll have to get creative with side streets to avoid heavy traffic on your way to South Park Drive. N.J. Transit bus 413 will drop you along North Park Drive, and of course, there is all kinds of parking here.

Food and Drink

You'll find picnic pavilions and benches every which way. The Lobster Trap is on the path, with other restaurants nearby on Marlton Pike.

Side Trip

If you haven't been mini golfing lately, there's a course on the corner of Cuthbert and Park Boulevard.

Where to Bike Rating

About...

The paved path around Cooper River is a terrific option for families – it's long enough for adults to enjoy and short enough for kids to tackle. The path runs about a mile and three quarters on either side of the river with two small bridges, and it is totally flat. You'll also find about a million other things to do here besides cycle!

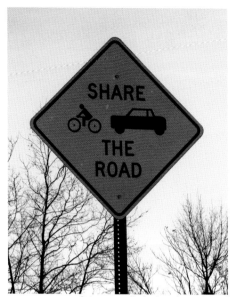

Drivers actually do share the roads here!

There is plenty of parking available here, so while the ride log begins at the lot off of Shady Lane and South Park Drive, you should feel free to hop on the path wherever you like. You don't have to worry about getting lost on this ride – just keep making right turns until you find your way back to where you began. And it's perfectly okay to bike along North and South Park drives if you want to ride a little bit faster.

The park provides 326 acres of playtime in the middle of Camden County, so the path is always full. The river itself is like a breath of fresh air. I visited the park in the winter while there was still snow on the ground and was happy to see cross-country skiers, joggers, and a few brave cyclists enjoying the river.

There are so many activities here in addition to cycling. On land, you can bring your mutt and play in the pooch park, enjoy one of the volleyball courts, visit the Sculpture Garden, or goof off in the huge playground. Cooper River also hosts free music festivals in the summer. If you want to bike and enjoy the water, there is a boat launch for sailing and fishing! Cooper River is also a major rowing destination, with crews practicing on the water and weekend regattas in season.

Additionally, you may see a bit of wildlife if you visit the river early enough in the morning. Red-bellied turtles, osprey, heron, geese and mallard live here. In the spring, migrant birds stop by the Cooper River as a little oasis – Yellow Warblers, Eastern Kingbirds, and Gray Catbirds are all about.

For more information about the bike path and all of the things to see and do here, visit www.camden-county.com/parks.

South Jersey

Ride Log

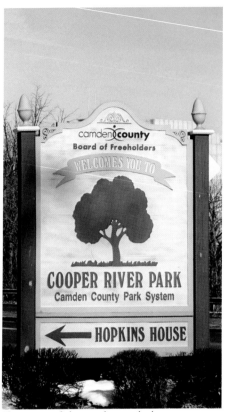

The winter sun feels so good on your back.

0.0 Begin at the parking lot by Shady Ln and South Park Dr. The Hopkins House Gallery of Contemporary Art will be to your right. Head left on the path or along South Park Dr.

0.2 Pass the Cooper River Yacht Club.

1.3 Make a right to head over the Cooper River.

1.5 Make another right to pick up the path, on the other side.

2.2 Pass the Camden County Boathouse.

2.6 North Park Dr becomes Park Blvd.

3.1 Take another right! Cross the Cooper River again, this time at Cuthbert Blvd.

3.3 Your final right turn! You will be back on S Park Dr heading towards Shady Ln.

3.8 And done. Let's do it again!

P1 Cooper River Yacht Club
P2 Camden County Boathouse
P3 Miniature Golf Course
P4 Hopkins Gallery

Cooper River Park

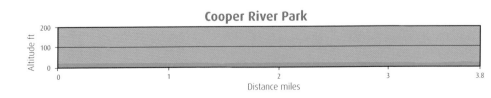

Altitude ft

Distance miles

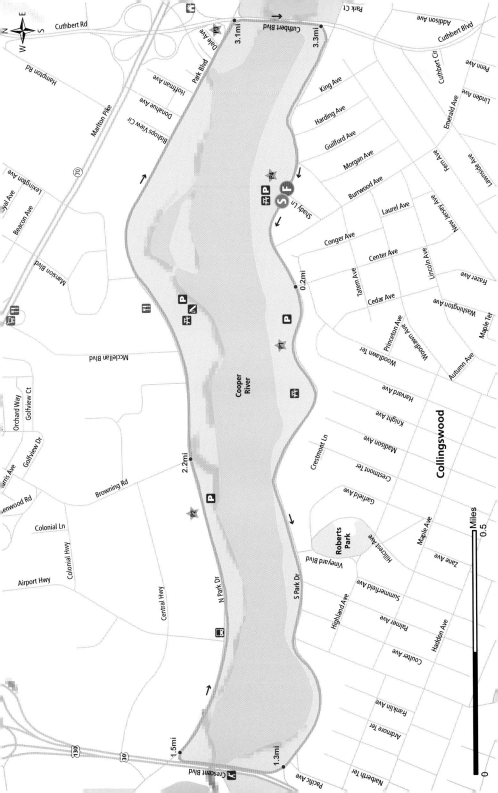

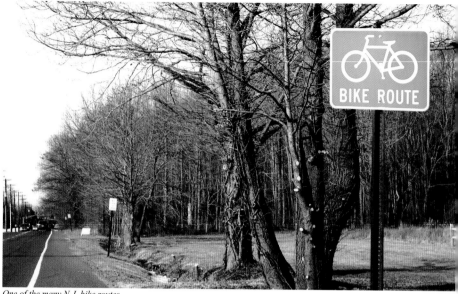

One of the many N.J. bike routes.

At a Glance

Distance 35.8 miles   **Total Elevation** 163 feet

Terrain

On road in South Jersey! You'll hit some little hills along the way, but for the most part, you'll enjoy long, even roads. A few straight aways will offer you lavish shoulders.

Traffic

You'll see steady traffic closer to Cherry Hill, but it dissipates by the time you hit the llama farm on the corner of Creek and Crispin roads. A few very big intersections (including Route 38 and Route 73) warrant caution.

How to Get There

You gotta drive! But there are more parking spaces at the starting point of this ride than the entire population of Cherry Hill could ever use.

Food and Drink

The big lunch/rest stop is at mile 20.5, on the corner of Marne Highway and Centerton Road, but be careful of the drivers in the parking lot of this huge strip mall!

Side Trip

The loop swings by the edge of the Rancocas State Park, which hosts two Juried American Indian Arts Festivals every year. There is also a small museum managed by the Powhatan Renape Nation and a replica of a traditional woodland village.

Links to

Where to Bike Rating

About...

This is the first of many long, luxurious rides though South Jersey! Dave Wender of the Outdoor Club of South Jersey provided me with this cue, which makes one big loop between Cherry Hill, Mt. Laurel, Cinnaminson and Riverton, with a monster lunch stop in between. This loop is a cool mix of town and country, and for nearly 40 miles, you'll have the pleasure of pedaling along some of the best roads South Jersey has to offer.

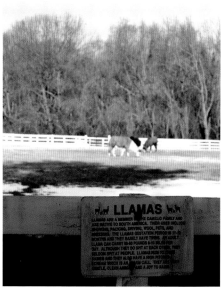

Llamas along the way.

Surprise! The ride log starts in a Corporate Park! The Woodland Falls Corporate Park, to be exact. It's located at the corner of New Jersey Route 38 and Mill Road. The best part about this starting point is suiting up and getting ready to ride while flaunting your freedom at those going inside to work.

The first bit of the ride will take you out of Cherry Hill along mostly residential roads. There are some busy intersections to watch out for – including Route 38. Just take your time and cross at the light.

Around mile five, you're in for some terrific straight ways – Elbo Lane, Hainesport/Mount Laurel, and Stacy Haines Road. They will take you out to the most rural portion of the ride, passing farmland, a few old barns, and eventually – the random llama yard on the corner of Crispin and Creek roads.

Keep on pedaling and before you know it, you'll hit the lunch stop on Marne Highway and Centerton. Dave planned the route perfectly – he knew you'd be starving by now! When you're finished with your break, hop back on Marne Highway and take a left onto Westfield. This can be a tricky intersection. You're headed in the right direction if the first cross street you encounter is Borton Landing Road.

You'll ride through Westfield, Riverton, and Cinnaminson before reaching the second most awesome spot on this ride (next to the llamas, of course); the intersection of Riverton and Bank streets. The first time I followed this route, I was blown away. The Delaware opens up before you, and out of nowhere you are treated to a stunning view of the river and the city.

After the river, you'll bike about six miles back to the corporate center, again on a mix of residential and commercial roads. Big intersections to beware of include routes 130, 73 and again at Route 38. But hey, I'll take those busy roads in exchange for Elbo, Stacy Haines, and Bank!

If you liked this route, check out Dave's other enjoyable cue: Cape May Lighthouse to Delaware Bay (Ride 49).

South Jersey

Ride Log

0.0 Start out at Woodland Falls Corporate Park and cross Rt 38 at the light. You'll be on West Mill Rd. Right on Fellowship Rd at the T, followed by a quick left onto Mill Rd (same intersection).

1.2 Left on Boulevard Ave at the T.

1.4 Right on Main St/Rt 537.

1.7 Right on Franklin Ave (turns into Grant, then Winthrop).

2.3 Right on Lenola Rd, then a quick left onto Westbrook Dr.

2.7 Cross Kings Hwy, pick up Haines Dr.

3.6 Right on Pleasant Valley Ave.

4.5 Right on Church St.

4.7 Left on Elbo Ln. If you hit Texas Ave, you've gone too far!

8.9 Elbo merges with Stacey Hines Rd – you're sure to enjoy this road!

11.4 Left on Fostertown Rd.

12.5 Right on Crispin Rd.

13.6 Left on Creek Rd. There's a llama farm on this corner!!

14.6 Left on Easton Way.

15.6 Right on Hainesport/Mt Laurel Rd. You're going to cross Rt 38 in a moment – use caution here.

16.1 Left on Creek Rd.

16.7 Left on Marne Hwy.

19.5 Lunch break! Take a left on Centerton Rd to visit the Centerton Shopping Center, which, in case you were curious, does in fact have a Chic-fil-A. If you're good to go, continue straight along Westfield Rd.

20.0 Cross Borton Landing Rd.

 P1 Strawbridge Park Bike Path
P2 Rancocas State Park, Hainesport, Burlington, New Jersey

 B1 EMS, 400 NJ 38, Moorestown, NJ 0857
B2 Mr Bill's, 9 West Broad St, Palmyra, NJ

21.8 Right on Haines Mill Rd.

22.5 Left of Tenby Chase Dr.

22.9 Left on Parry Rd.

23.8 Right on Winding Brook Dr.

24.0 Left on Wayne Dr.

25.0 Right on Riverton Rd, pedal here for the next two miles.

26.9 Right on Howard St.

27.3 Left on Bank Ave – ooooh lovely views of the Delaware!

28.0 Left at Cinnaminson Ave.

28.2 Right at Temple Blvd (flashing yellow).

28.7 Left on Jefferson St.

28.9 Left on Market St.

29.2 Cross Broad St.

29.9 Bear left on Fairfax Dr.

30.2 Right on Cinnaminson.

31.0 Right on Lenola Rd at the light.

31.3 Right on Fork Landing Rd. Use caution when crossing Rt 73 up ahead.

33.5 Cross Main St/Rt 573.

34.2 Right on Mill Rd, cross Rt 38.

35.8 And back to the lot!

Dave's Cherry Hill Loop

Altitude ft / Distance miles

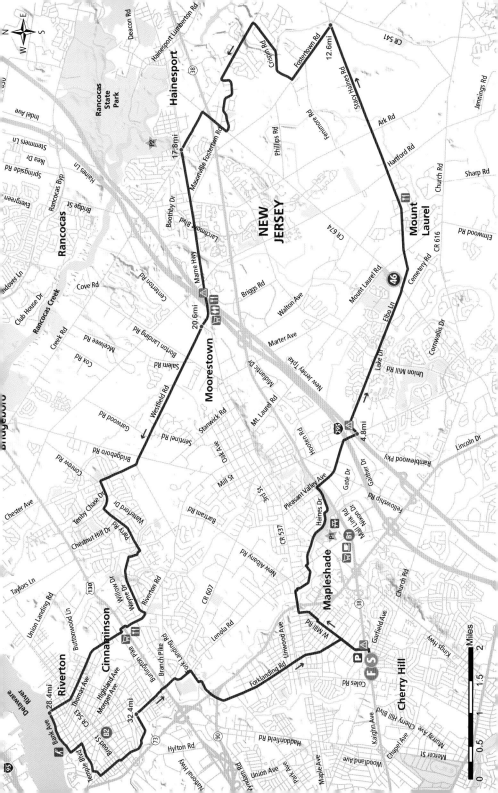

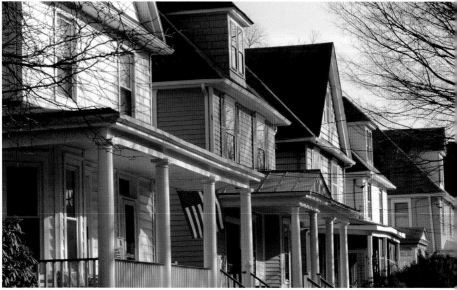

Lovely Haddonfield.

At a Glance

Distance 3.5 miles   **Total Elevation** 111 feet

Terrain

It's just so flat! You'll be pedaling along enjoyable, residential roads on your maiden PATCO voyage.

Traffic

Aside from the time you're riding on Haddon Avenue in both Collingswood and Haddonfield, and the block of Kings Highway in Haddonfield, the roads will be quiet to traffic and full of speed bumps to keep the cars moving slowly through the neighborhoods.

How to Get There

Hop on the PATCO from Center City! A round trip ticket from Philadelphia to the Haddonfield and Collingswood stations will cost you under $5.

Food and Drink

Both Collingswood and Haddonfield have numerous cafés, restaurants and pizza shops for you to enjoy, and in the warmer months, you'll have your pick of outdoor dining. Check out Haddon Avenue in Collingswood and Kings Highway in Haddonfield.

Side Trip

Aside from enjoying all that these towns have to offer, you should probably visit the statue of the Hadrosaurus (The official state dinosaur of New Jersey) in the center of Haddonfield. It's true! Then visit the bountiful Farmer's Market across the street (in season).

Where to Bike Rating

About...

Restless? Tired of city streets? Hop on the PATCO for a quick change of pace! This one-way ride is just under four miles, and my oh my, will it remind you of bygone days tooling streets as a kiddo. This ride also makes for a great date ride – there's little exertion, you'll feel like you're far from the city, and there are plenty of romantic restaurants. Plus, you can always ride back to Collingswood for a cool 7.5 mile loop.

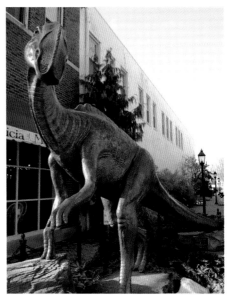

The Haddonfield Hadrosaurus.

You'll never be far from Haddon Avenue, or a PATCO station, on this one way tour through the 'burbs of Collingswood and Haddonfield. It's perfect for a slow, suburban bike ride.

Collingswood has a big arts community, which celebrates with new exhibitions on second Saturdays. There's also a few annual art festivals, a book festival, and two theater companies! There are over 20 restaurants and even more shops squeezed into its central district on Haddon Avenue.

You may want to give this ride a try if you are a novice, as the roads are very easy to follow and with little traffic. If riding near cars scares you, then feel free to walk your bike through Collingswood and hop on at the Lincoln Avenue turn. Likewise, hop off your bike on Haddon Avenue in Haddonfield and walk yourself down Kings Highway.

If you are a more experienced rider, you might enjoy this jaunt on a sunny afternoon with a couple of friends and a long, relaxed lunch in between pedaling and PATCOing. It's very low-stress riding, and the cue has under 15 turns.

When you reach Haddonfield, you might want to walk around the shops and restaurants on Kings Highway and Haddon Avenue, or time your ride to catch Fall Festival in October or the Haddonfield Crafts & Fine Arts Festival in the summer. There's a small historical preservation district here to explore too – Haddonfield was founded by Elizabeth Haddon in the early 18th century, after she arrived from England in 1701. Be sure to stop by the Indian King Tavern historical site and museum – noted for its unique role in the American Revolution.

When you're ready to head home, hop on PATCO back to the city at Haddonfield or ride on back to Collingswood. Either way, this is a great afternoon ride for you and your slow bicycle.

South Jersey

Ride Log

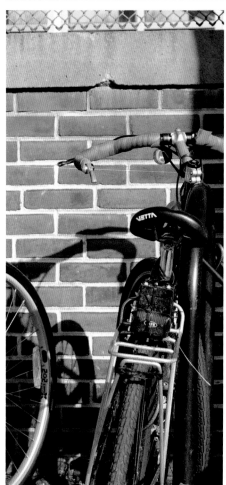

Bicycles waiting for Patco.

0.0 Start out at the Collingswood PATCO station. Exit station on Haddon Ave, and make a left. The first cross street will be Frazer Ave.

0.3 You'll ride through the heart of Collingswood, and then make a right on Lincoln Ave.

0.4 A quick right on Maple Ave.

1.0 Left at the T intersection on Penn Ave.

1.1 Take the next right. It will be Oriental Ave.

1.4 Left on Cambridge Ave at the T-intersection.

1.5 Take the next right – it's pretty quick! – onto Virginia Ave.

1.9 Right on Locust Ave, then a quick left onto Elm Ave.

2.1 Left on Maple Ave at the T-intersection.

2.3 Right onto Wood Ln.

2.8 Right on Hopkins Ave.

3.0 Make a right onto N Haddon Ave. This road will have steady traffic.

3.2 Right onto Clement St followed by a quick left (at the T) on Tanner St.

3.3 Right onto Kings Hwy (again busier than most of the other streets on this ride!)

3.5 Right into the Haddonfield PATCO station. Lock up your bikes and have a walk around!

P1 Hadrosaurus Statue
P2 Farmers Market (in season)

B1 Freeride Sports, 8 King's Highway East, Haddonfield, NJ

Back Roads from Collingswood to Haddonfield

Altitude ft / Distance miles

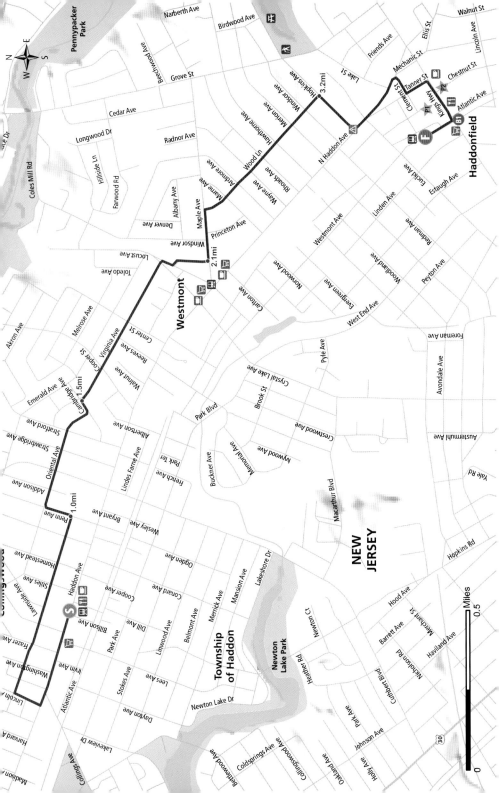

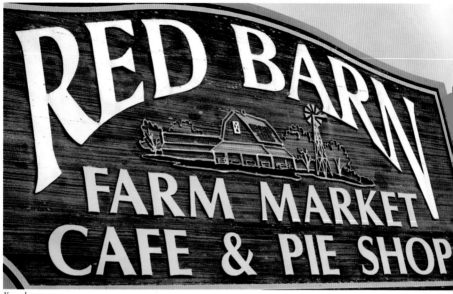

Yes, please.

At a Glance

Distance 51.4 miles   **Total Elevation** 188 feet

Terrain

All flat, all on road. You'll enjoy wide shoulders and a bike route or two as well. The ride mixes residential and commercial streets with vast rural landscapes.

Traffic

Most of this ride is quiet, however, there are a few streets that will have steady traffic, and some will be fast – especially Route 206.

How to Get There

Driving is your best bet. Medford is about 40 minutes away from Philadelphia on Route 70, and there is ample parking at the start point at St. Peter's Church on Christopher Mill Road.

Food and Drink

Hammonton, which is about half way through the ride, has numerous cafés and snack shops. The Red Barn,

the namesake of this ride, has the best pie in South Jersey. It is a couple of miles north of downtown, and is a must!

Side Trip

Take a quick dip! Nestled in Wharton State Forest on Route 206, the Atsion Recreation Area is open all summer long for swimming and relaxing.

Links to 46 47

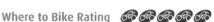

Where to Bike Rating

About...

If you love bicycling and baked goods as much as I do, then this loop will be an instant favorite! Enjoy the long, flat roads of South Jersey from Medford to Hammonton, stop by the Red Barn for a piece of pie and some extra energy, then pedal home through Wharton State Forest. This tried and true route comes to us from the Outdoor Club of South Jersey – thanks to them for sharing this tradition!

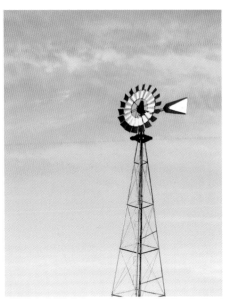

Red Barn beckons!

According to Jeff Thomas of the OCSJ, there are many varieties of the Pie Ride, but this is one of the original routes (an off-shoot of the Friday morning cue led by Fran Horn). According to Jeff "I named this ride Pie a la Mode since the Red Barn has the best pie in South Jersey (they also have the best muffins; but , who wants to go on a ride called the Muffin Ride?). Good point. Thanks also to Dolly Bernard for helping me to track down the route!

With its beautiful farmland, the twists and turns of Pie Ride a la Mode will help you remember why they call it the Garden State. You'll start in a familiar place in Medford – the starting points for Rides 46 and 47 are just up the road – and head down long stretches of comfortable cycling roads towards more scenic landscapes. The cue takes advantage of a few bike routes as well – the kind of well marked extended shoulder only present in South Jersey.

Some of the long wonderful roads you will encounter: Kettle Run for four and a half miles, Old White Horse Pike for five miles, and Atsion for six and a half. These roads are among the longest straight aways in this book, and they provide an excellent backdrop for tandem riding and good conversation.

Now, a few of the turns are tricky. Some of the roads are marked with teeny signs, and one or two I couldn't find at all. There are two tiny roads to watch out for specifically – Ehrke at mile 19.2 and Midbridge at 44.8. You've passed Ehrke if you find yourself at the intersection of Route 30 and Route 143, and you've passed Midbridge if you hit Wigwam Court, and you've really passed it if you hit Tuckerton Road.

Hammonton is at mile 28 and is a great place to stop for lunch or stretch your legs. After Hammonton, you'll make your way up Bellevue Avenue/Route 54 and pick up Trenton Road/Route 206. Use caution on Route 206 – the cars will be moving pretty fast. Red Barn is at mile marker two of Route 206 on the left. Look out for the windmill up ahead!

After pie, you'll take Atsion back towards Medford, wind through a few residential streets and then arrive again at St. Peter's. On your return, your first thought will be that second slice of pie you should have had!

South Jersey

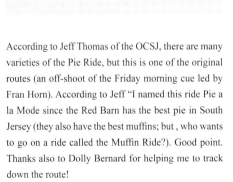

Ride Log

0.0 Start at St Peter's Church in Medford on the corner of Christopher Mill Rd and Taunton Rd. Make a right on Christopher Mill, away from Taunton.

1.6 Right onto Tuckerton Rd, pick up the bike route. Tuckerton becomes E Main St.

3.1 Left on S Elmswood Rd.

4.2 Left on Tomlinson Mill Rd.

5.0 Make a slight left to pick up Kettle Run. Stick here for the next 4.6 miles, following street signs at the forks.

9.6 Right at Hopewell Rd (T-intersection).

10.3 Left on Raymond Ave.

11.3 Right on Cooper Rd.

12.4 Left on Granger Ave.

12.5 Right on Atco Ave.

12.9 Come to a funny intersection with Hayes Mill Rd. Take the very sharp left onto Hayes Mill.

13.4 Left on Cooper Folly Rd. Cross Rt 30.

13.9 Right on W Atlantic Ave, which turns into Old White Horse Pike.

19.2 Right on Ehrke Rd (it is small, just before the large intersection with Rt 143 and Rt 30). You'll cross Rt 30 again while on Ehrke.

20.5 Left on Waterford Rd.

20.9 Left on Cedar St.

21.7 Left on E Central Ave.

22.8 Right on Rt 143.

24.9 Left on County Rd 561/ S Egg Harbor Rd.

28.8 You'll reach Hammonton. Cross the train tracks and make a left onto Rt 54/Bellevue Ave – the main street through Hammonton.

29.9 Slight right to stay on Bellevue Ave and cross Rt 30.

30.0 Pick up Rt 206/Trenton Rd and head North. Pie in less than two miles!

31.8 Red Barn Café! You'll be at mile marker two on Rt 206. Post-pie, hop back on your ride and take a left on 206 to head towards Wharton State Forest. Stick on 206 for the next six or so miles.

37.3 Left on Atsion Rd.

44.8 Left at Midbridge Dr into the residential streets.

45.5 Right at Highbridge Blvd.

46.4 Left on Gravelly Hollow Rd, which becomes Fairview Rd.

48.9 Right on Chestnut Rd, continue on E Lake Blvd.

49.8 Left at Falls Rd.

49.9 Right at Taunton Blvd.

51.4 Left on Christopher Mill to reach your start point. Whew!

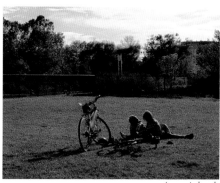

A pre-pie break.

 P1 Penza's Pies at the Red Barn, South Myrtle Street, Hammonton, NJ

 P2 Atsion Recreation Area

B B1 Pro Pedals Bike Shop, 682 White Horse Pike, Hammonton, NJ

Pie Ride a la Mode

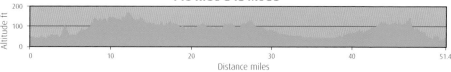

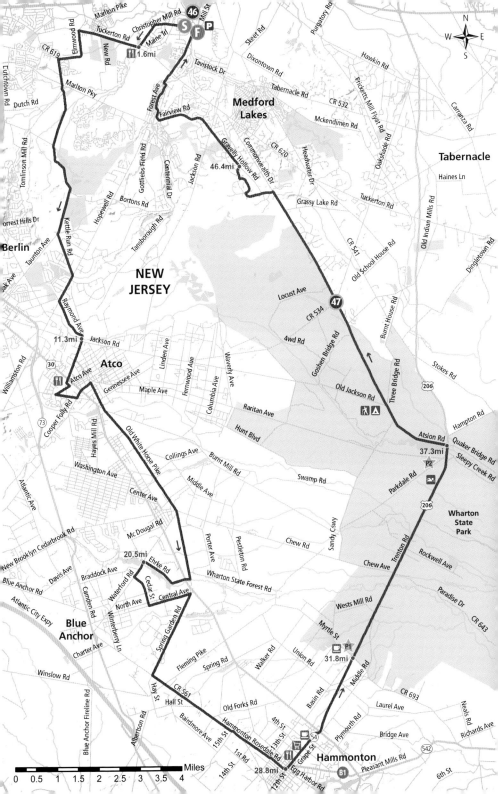

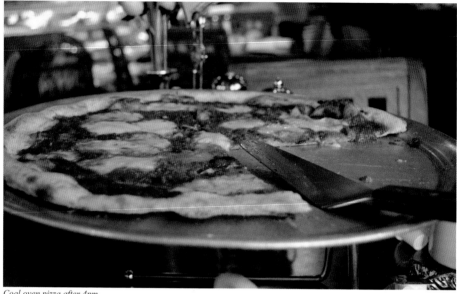

Coal oven pizza after 4pm.

At a Glance

Distance 42.8 miles   **Total Elevation** 113 feet

Terrain

The route to the Olde World Bakery is all on-road riding with long, flat stretches of bicycle lanes.

Traffic

A mix – some roads have steady traffic, others very little. All will have famously long New Jersey yellow lights.

How to Get There

This ride, along with 47, starts at the Taunton Forge shopping area at the intersection of Taunton Boulevard and Tuckerton Road in Medford, New Jersey. It's about a 30 minute drive from Philadelphia along Route 70, with tons of parking.

Food and Drink

You'll want to have a pizza or a snack at the excellent Olde World Bakery. There are a few places along the way to grab a drink in a pinch, but, let's be real here, nothing compares to fresh baked goods in the middle of a 42.8 mile loop. A word to the wise; brick oven pizza only available after 4:30pm, so plan this ride on a long summer day.

Side Trip

A stop by Johnson's Corner Farm on Church Road is a nice way to begin or end your day – there is a farmstand, bakery and pick-your-own strawberries, blueberries, peaches, sweet corn, apples, and best for biking – pumpkins!

Links to 43 45 47

Where to Bike Rating

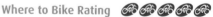

About...

A big thank you to Joe Racite, ride leader for the Tri-County Cyclists, for this cue out to the Olde World Bakery (a favorite rest stop amongst South Jersey cyclists). You'll be delighted by the number of bicycle lanes you'll encounter along the way, as well as the relatively good bicycle to car culture–you won't be honked at as much as in the city, and drivers will even let you have the right of way from time to time!

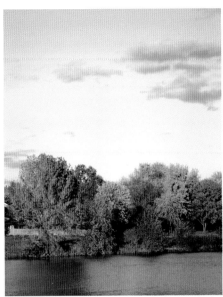

Have a rest by the water's edge.

The route to the Olde World Bakery is similar to other South Jersey rides – it is long and flat and includes a lot of streets whose names sort of sound the same. There are a few luxurious stretches that will invite you to pedal harder and faster than usual, because you won't be hitting a traffic light for as far as the eye can see.

This ride was my first in South Jersey, and I have to admit that I was really surprised by the beauty and calming sensation on some of these roads (not all, of course, there were plenty of mini-vans and SUVs to contend with along the way). The route is a simple figure eight with 27 miles of riding before you reach the bakery and 15 after. If you like this cue but want a shorter distance, try Ride 47 by the same dude: Joe's Ride to Nixon's General Store.

The beginning of this ride is probably the most confusing. It will likely take you a few tries to get yourself properly oriented if you're new to the area. The goal is to head north on Taunton Road, and you'll know you're on the right track when you cross Holly Road. If you see Falls Road, turn that bike around and head in the opposite direction!

Most of the roads out to the bakery are excellent for the kind of meditative cycling where you get lost in the rhythm of the cadence. The landscape will jump back and forth between suburban and rural, and the roads go on and on for days. Fostertown, in my opinion, is one of the best roads for cycling in the area. Other very frequently traveled roads for South Jersey cyclists include Church Road, Eayestown Road, Stacey-Haines Road, and Hainsport-Mt Laurel Road.

It was a real pleasure to take this ride in the fall when the foliage was incredible and the pumpkin patches were in full swing. But I intend to head out there again in the summer, and probably every summer from now on, to pick blueberries and enjoy this gorgeous part of New Jersey. And scarf another Margherita pizza from Olde World. They're delicious.

South Jersey

Ride Log

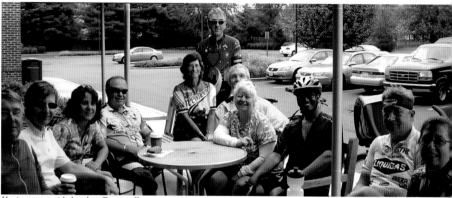

Having a post ride lunch at Taunton Forge.

P1 Johnson Family Farm,
133 Church Rd, Medford, NJ
P2 Olde World Bakery, 1000 Smithville Road,
Mount Holly, NJ
P3 Medford Park

B1 Wheelies Bike Shop, 176 Route 70,
Suite 6A, Malrton NJ
B2 Mt Holly Schwinn Bicycles, 1645 NJ 38,
Mt Holly, NJ

0.0 Start out on Taunton Blvd and Tuckerton Rd heading north on Taunton Rd. Holly Rd is the first cross street in the correct direction, Falls Rd is the first intersection in the incorrect direction.

1.4 Bear left on Hartford Rd.

4.0 Make a left on Church Rd at Johnson's Farm Rd.

7.6 Make a hard right on Hainesport/Mt Laurel Rd. Pedal along Hainesport for the next five miles.

12.6 Right on Fostertown Rd – caution! The sign for Fostertown was itty bitty when I was mapping this route.

17.2 Left on Church Rd at the T-intersection.

19.6 Left on Eayrestown Rd. This sounds funny, but there are two Eayerstown roads – you are looking for the second.

21.6 Right on Newbolds-Corner Rd.

23.3 Left on Smithville Rd. Cross Rt 38.

27.8 Right on Woodlane Rd. You've reached the Olde World Bakery! After your rest and pizza, head out the way you came – back down Smithville Rd.

30.5 Right on Newbold - Corner Rd

32.1 Cross Eayrestown Rd and pedal straight to Municipal Dr.

33.4 Left on Main St/ Rt 541.

35.0 Right on Fostertown Rd.

35.2 A quick left on Stacy Haines Rd.

37.6 Left on Hartford, heading back towards Johnson's farm.

41.3 Bear right to pick up Taunton Blvd.

42.8 Arrive at Taunton Forge!

The Olde World Bakery

Altitude ft

Distance miles

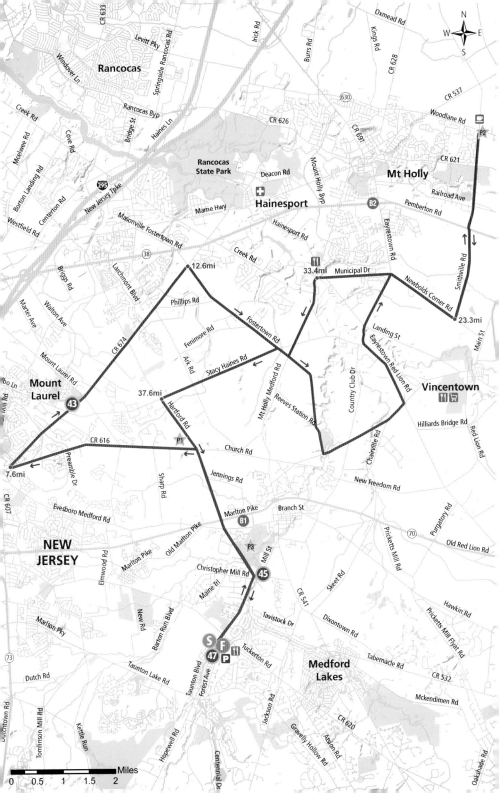

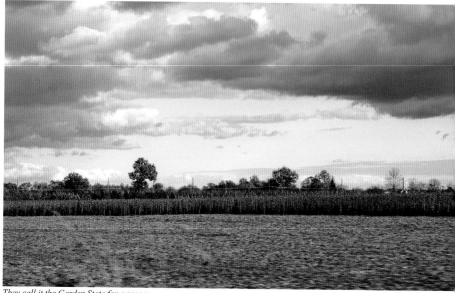

They call it the Garden State for a reason.

At a Glance

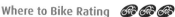

Distance 22.5 miles   **Total Elevation** 164 feet

Terrain

You'll pedal along flat, tree lined and rural roads on your way to Nixon's.

Traffic

Some roads will have more traffic than others, but there are beautifully wide New Jersey shoulders on almost all the roads which accommodate cyclists nicely.

How to Get There

This ride, along with Ride 46, starts at the Taunton Forge shopping area at the intersection of Taunton Boulevard and Tuckerton Road in Medford, New Jersey. It's about a 30 minute drive from Philadelphia along Route 70, with tons of parking.

Food and Drink

Eat a delicious deli sandwich at Nixon's. It is another favorite rest stop for South Jersey cyclists. There are picnic tables outside and rocking chairs on the porch. You'll want to stay a while!

Side Trip

You'll pass the Wharton State Park on Atsion Road – lock up the bikes and take a walk through the pines to stretch out your legs. There are rivers and creeks every which way, and the further in you venture, the more likely you'll be to see ospreys, hawks, herons, and swans, among other birds and wildlife.

Links to 45 46

Where to Bike Rating

About...

The trip out to Nixon's is a great introduction to the sumptuous roads of South Jersey – you'll take just a few turns, pedal through both suburban and rural patches, and push the pace along some of those killer straight-aways. The ride log is very straight forward, so for those unfamiliar with the area, you needn't worry too much about getting turned around. And then, a cold drink and sandwich await you at Nixon's!

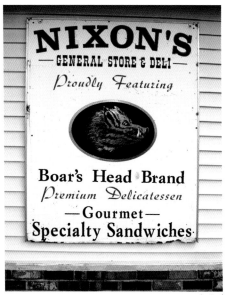

Arrive!

As with Ride 46, the beginning of this ride is the most confusing. It might take you a few tries to become properly oriented if you're new to the area. The goal is to head east on Tuckerton Road. You'll be heading in the correct direction if you pass Ashley Court/Oakwood Drive, and in the very wrong direction if you hit Maine Trail or Christopher Mill Road.

You'll pedal along the shady Tuckerton for the first five miles, if you've successfully negotiated the start. Take advantage of the shoulder here and go at your own pace – these roads suit a variety of riding styles. You can meander along or burn it up.

There are only about four turns on this log (five if you count turning around at Nixon's), meaning there is ample time for spacing out and letting your mind wander. Just don't miss a turn!

Once you hit Oakshade, there will be a bit more open space. To head towards Nixon's make a left. If you want to cut the ride short, make a right on Oakshade and pick up the ride log at mile 13.8. This will give you a 16.2 mile loop, and you can still grab lunch at Taunton Forge.

If you are doing the full loop to Nixon's, then you'll pedal down Oakshade for about two miles and then Medford Lakes for about two more. If you want to extend the ride from 22 to 42 miles, and have a taste of the Pine Barrens, then take Chatsworth Road to Tabernacle-Chatsworth Road (bearing right) to Main Street in Chatsworth (this is Joe's original route). You'll come back along the same roads and pick up the ride log at 9.5.

The way back from Nixon's is a little bit different – you'll stay on Oakshade and pedal past Tuckerton on your way to Atsion Road, which is another great cycling stretch. Atsion eventually merges with Tuckerton and brings you back to the starting point.

Another big thank you to Joe Racite, ride leader for the Tri-County Cyclists, for this cue. If you like this ride, check out Joe's other, longer route, Ride 46: The Olde World Bakery.

South Jersey

Ride Log

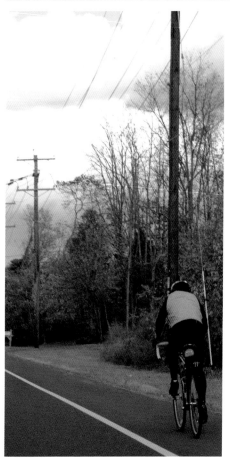

A lovely autumn bicycle ride.

0.0 Start at the corner of Taunton Blvd and Tuckerton Rd. Head East on Tuckerton. The first cross street will be Oakwood Dr/Ashley Ct.

1.3 Cross Jackson Rd.

4.0 Cross Stokes Rd.

5.5 Left on Oakshade Rd. If you hit Rt 206, you've gone too far.

7.8 Right on Medford Lakes Rd.

9.5 Cross Carranza Rd. Nixon's is up ahead on the left. Have a rest! Grab a sandwich! When you're all set, start pedaling back down Medford Lakes in the direction you came from.

11.3 Left on Oakshade Rd.

13.8 Cross Tuckerton Rd.

15.8 Right on Atsion (Connector with Ride 45: Pie Ride a la Mode).

20.8 Left on Tuckerton Rd.

22.5 Arrive back at Taunton and Tuckerton roads.

 P1 Nixon's General Store,
540 Chatsworth Rd, Tabernacle NJ

Joe's Ride to Nixon's General Store

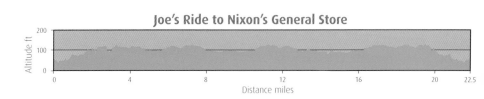

Altitude ft

Distance miles

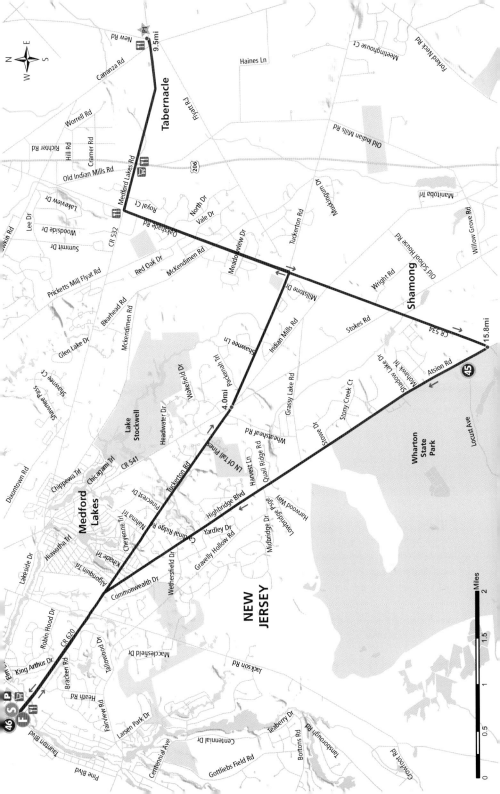

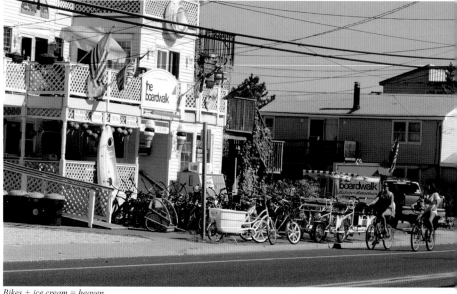

Bikes + ice cream = heaven.

At a Glance

Distance 38.1 miles   **Total Elevation** 18 feet

Terrain

You'll really enjoy riding on this barrier island – it is super flat and super fast. There are also loads of bike lanes and bike friendly side streets.

Traffic

There is room for everyone on this popular island. Bike lanes in Beach Haven are more crowded with families and kiddos than some of the other sections of the island, but you'll find plenty of room for passing. Traffic on Long Beach Boulevard is steady; you may want to consider taking a quieter side street if you don't love racing cars to the lights.

How to Get There

If driving from Philadelphia, head east until you hit the water. There is one bridge to bring you on and off the island. You'll find parking all over, but the ride log starts at the south end of the island.

Food and Drink

Make sure you work up an appetite for all of the excellent Jersey Shore food that awaits your empty landlocked belly. There are ice cream shops every few blocks, including Kelly's at the turnaround. For pizza and fries, Bay Village in Beach Haven is the best. Hit the Shell for a cold beer poolside.

Side Trip

Take a dip in the Atlantic!

Where to Bike Rating

About...

Long Beach Island makes for the perfect cycling getaway. The barrier island is 18 miles long and just a few blocks wide – meaning you can almost always see both the bay and the ocean. There are quiet side streets, loads of bike lanes, and one very fast boulevard. You will pass kids riding with surfboards, grandmas in sun hats, tiny tykes on training wheels, spandex clad club riders and just about everyone else on two wheels. Plus there are bicycle shops and rentals all over the island to help you on your way.

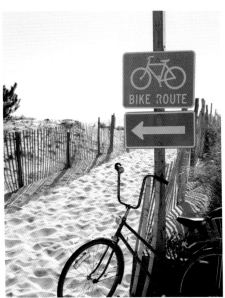

My summer ride.

Long Beach Island is another huge favorite of mine. The hour and a half drive from Philadelphia is worth every minute whether you go during the busy and warm summer months or the relaxed and lovely autumn.

The ride log begins at the south end of the island in Holgate, and it is very simple. You will ride north until you reach the lighthouse, or get pooped out, and then you'll turn around and ride south. In general, you will always have the option of bike lanes or a quiet side street, and when it comes time to cross the boulevard (which separates the ocean side from the bay side), you will find signs on the side streets indicating which blocks have traffic lights.

There is one hairy section with more traffic than others, and that is the area near the bridge. While drivers are very used to bicycles on the island, it would do you good to ride with a bit more caution in this area – there are some awkward one-ways and you'll have to ride on the boulevard for a bit.

If you do choose to ride the full length of the island, you will be greeted in the north by the iconic red and white lighthouse known as Ol' Barney. There is a small state park where you can stretch your legs and learn about Barney's history. You'll also find a few casual restaurants nearby, an ice cream shop, and some fun kitshy shops.

You will get the lay of the land quickly and feel very comfortable exploring the island on your own, but the naming convention of the cross streets might make you nuts. There are eight different towns that make up LBI, and so the numbered cross streets go up and down again and up again and sometimes skip entire groups of numbers, and the name of the main boulevard changes here and there.

My advice is to go ahead and make a weekend out of it – there is plenty of lodging available and even more of what we all really want out of life: kayak rentals, ice cream, and mini golf. If you have to make a quick turnaround, then stop into the Sandbox Café & Bath House in Ship Bottom for a bite and a rinse.

The traffic lights on the boulevard switch to flashing yellows after the annual Chowderfest in September, which, depending on your riding style, you will either love or hate!

South Jersey

Ride Log

0.0 Start in the bike lanes at the southern tip of the island. Head north.

1.6 Make a right onto Liberty Ave.

1.7 Follow the arrow to pick up the bike lanes on Beach Ave.

2.0 Right on Dolphin Ave.

2.1 Left on Atlantic Ave.

3.3 The lane narrows.

4.3 Left on 34th St at the T, then a right on Beach Ave.

4.9 Right on 121st St and left on Beach. Stay straight for a ways.

8.6 Left on 31st St. Take note: If you don't want to touch Long Beach Blvd, then turn yourself right around and head home. You'll still have a 17 mile ride on your hands.

8.7 If you don't mind the traffic, then make a right onto Long Beach Blvd.

8.8 Left on 26th St at the light. You'll be on the bay side of the island now.

8.9 Right on Central Ave. Nice shoulder here!

9.6 You might not like this – make a right at 11th St.

9.7 Left back onto Long Beach Blvd. Make sure you get all the way over to the right – you are close to the lone bridge and there is high traffic here. Stay on Long Beach Blvd through to Surf City.

10.4 Left at the light on Third St –Scojo's diner is on the corner.

10.5 Right on Central Ave.

11.5 Right on 23rd St.

11.6 Left back on Long Beach Blvd – yahooooo bike lanes are back in North Beach!

18.3 At Eighth St, bear left on the diagonal road. Follow the signs to Barnegat Lighthouse. Pass Rick's American Café and Kelly's Old Barney Restaurant.

18.7 Right through the entrance to Barnegat Lighthouse State Park…aka Ol' Barney.

18.8 When you're ready turn 'em around to head home!

18.9 Left back on Eighth St diagonal.

19.2 Right on Central Ave.

19.3 Quick right on Ninth St.

19.5 Left on Bayview Ave.

20.9 Left on Long Beach Blvd.

26.3 Right on 24th St.

26.4 Right on Central Ave.

28.0 Stay on Central Ave as you cross Rt. 72 – the road that leads to the bridge. High traffic area! Respect the stoplights!

29.0 Left on 28th St.

29.1 If you like riding with the traffic, then make a right on Long Beach Blvd. Fly down this road all the way to Nardi's! If that sounds like a bad idea to you, then make a left onto 31st St to pick up the ocean side bike lanes.

32.7 Left at Nardi's on 19th St.

32.8 Right on Beach Ave. Follow the curve and make a quick left to stick on the Southbound Beach Ave bike lanes.

34.7 Right on Taylor Ave and cross Long Beach Blvd. Pass Bay Village Pizza!

34.8 Left on Delaware Ave. No bike lanes but very quiet.

35.6 Right on Long Beach Blvd. Pearl Street Market is on the corner.

35.7 Right on Berkeley then a left onto West Ave.

36.7 Left on Nelson Ave.

36.8 Right on Long Beach Blvd bike lanes through Holgate.

38.1 Back to the start!

Long Beach Island Loop

Altitude ft / Distance miles

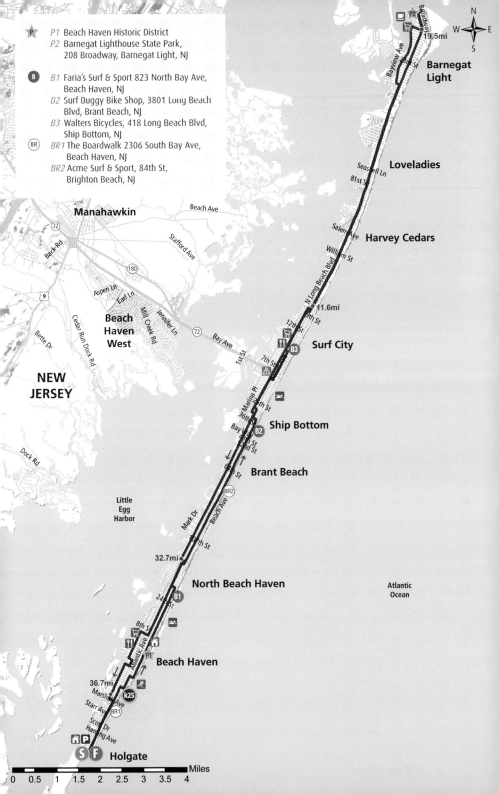

P1 Beach Haven Historic District
P2 Barnegat Lighthouse State Park,
208 Broadway, Barnegat Light, NJ

B1 Faria's Surf & Sport 823 North Bay Ave,
Beach Haven, NJ
B2 Surf Buggy Bike Shop, 3801 Long Beach
Blvd, Brant Beach, NJ
B3 Walters Bicycles, 418 Long Beach Blvd,
Ship Bottom, NJ

BR1 The Boardwalk 2306 South Bay Ave,
Beach Haven, NJ
BR2 Acme Surf & Sport, 84th St,
Brighton Beach, NJ

Barnegat
Light

19.5mi

Broadway

Bayview Ave

20th St

Loveladies

Seashell Ln

81st St

Harvey Cedars

Salem Ave

William St

N Long Beach Blvd

11.6mi

9th St

12th St

Surf City

7th St

B3

Beach Ave

Manahawkin

72

Stafford Ave

Back Rd

180

Aspen Ln

Earl Ln

Jennifer Ln

72

9

Cedar Run Dock Rd

Mill Creek Rd

Beach
Haven
West

1st St

Bay Ave

Bette Dr

NEW
JERSEY

Marina Pl

30th St

36th St

Ship Bottom

Bay Blvd

B2

32nd St

Dock Rd

Brant Beach

Little
Egg
Harbor

BR2

Beach Ave

Mark Dr

60th St

32.7mi

77th St

North Beach Haven

Atlantic
Ocean

24th St

B1

8th St

Atlantic Ave

Beach Haven

P1

36.7mi

Marshall Ave

25

Starr Ave

BR1

Scott Dr

Harding Ave

S F Holgate

Miles

0   0.5   1   1.5   2   2.5   3   3.5   4

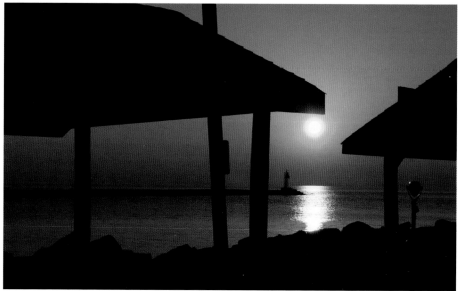

Sunset on Delaware Bay.

At a Glance

Distance 25.3 miles   **Total Elevation** 50 feet

Terrain

You're pedaling from the ocean to the bay – it doesn't get much flatter than this! Beach roads with bicycle lanes and long county roads make up the bulk of this ride.

Traffic

There is steady traffic all over the Jersey shore in the summer, and Cape May is no exception. It can be fun to ride along in the heat of August, but if you prefer cycling with less company, then try this one out in the spring or autumn to beat the crowds.

How to Get There

The drive to Cape May is just under two hours from Philadelphia via the Atlantic City Expressway and Garden State Parkway, so plan to leave early and spend a full day there or enjoy a lazy ride and spend the weekend at the shore. Depending on where you're coming from, it might also be possible to patch together Septa and N.J. Transit to get yourself to the center of town.

Food and Drink

You can't throw a dog in Cape May without hitting a beachy restaurant or snack shop. There are lots of great places to try, including an abundance of ice cream, pizza, and breakfast spots.

Side Trip

Go to the Cape May Zoo! There are zebras, lions, tigers and giraffes! And it's free everyday!

Where to Bike Rating

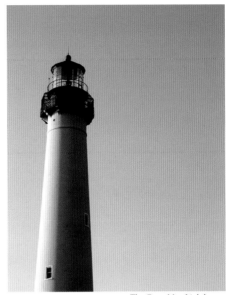

The Cape May Lighthouse.

About...

Cape May is beautiful! The brightly colored Victorian homes, coupled with one of the best beaches around, will keep you swooning all afternoon. This route will show you all the ins and outs of the area, as you crisscross the southern tip of New Jersey from the ocean to the bay. A big thanks to David Wender for suggesting this excellent ride!

You may want to start or end your day by having a look around the historic Cape May Lighthouse, which was built by the Army Corps of Engineers in 1859. It was automated in 1946, and it is still operational. The lighthouse park is open daily in the spring, summer and fall, and on weekends in the winter.

The first portion of this route brings you from the lighthouse to the center of town and all along the shoreline. You'll enjoy many of the bike lanes that Cape May has to offer, and in season, the company of all the other folks on two wheels.

One of the best portions of this ride happens early on – the stretch along Beach Drive. You'll pedal right alongside the ocean, and though it can be congested in certain places in the summer, it's a fun place to bike. Plus you can always jump in the water for a quick dip!

You'll wind through some of the suburban roads around Cape May as you head on Seashore Road towards the bridge over the inlet. The bridge might be intimidating at first, but just follow the bicycle signs and you'll be good to go.

After pedaling north for about three more miles after the bridge, you'll make a left on Breakwater Road and head west towards the Bay. Around mile 16, you'll

be almost there! I caught an awesome sunset here, and then popped on my lights for the ride home (might not be advisable, but it turned out pretty well for me).

The way home is pretty straightforward but there is one spot that is tricky – the turn onto New England Road/Route 641 after you cross back over the bridge. It is a really quick right at the bottom of the bridge – keep your eyes open for it! Otherwise you'll be good to go on your way back to the lighthouse.

One word to the wise: a lot of these roads have small street name signs, but are clearly marked by the route number, so where possible I tried to include both. A word to the wiser: Cape May is another beach tag town.

South Jersey

Ride Log

0.0 Start at Cape May Lighthouse parking area, exit on Lighthouse Ave.

0.3 Make a right on Seagrove Ave.

0.7 Right on Sunset Blvd/Rt 606.

1.9 Right on Broadway/Rt 626.

2.2 Left on Beach Dr/Rt 604 – ride along the ocean!

3.9 Left on Pittsburgh Ave/Rt622.

4.6 Left on Delaware Ave.

4.9 Left on Indiana Ave, then bear right on Michigan Ave.

5.3 Left on Madison Ave, and a very quick right on Columbia Ave.

5.7 Right on Ocean St (becomes Elmira St/Leaming Ave).

6.6 Right on Broadway/Seashore Rd/Rt 626.

8.0 Over the bridge!

11.1 Left on Breakwater Rd/Rt 613.

12.9 Right on Fishing Creek Rd/Rt 639.

13.4 Right on Bayshore Rd/Rt 603 at the light.

14.1 Left at Village Rd.

14.7 Left on Bay Dr.

16.0 Right on Pinewood Dr.

16.2 Left on Shore Dr – ride along the bay!

16.5 Left on Rosehill Pkwy.

18.5 Right on Bayshore Rd/Rt 603.

18.8 Bear left on Jonathan Hoffman Rd/Rt 603.

19.8 Bear left on Seashore Rd and follow signs towards the bridge.

20.1 Right on Rt 626 towards Cape May Bridge.

20.6 Make a quick right at the bottom of the bridge onto New England Rd/Rt 641.

21.6 Left on Stevens St.

 P1 Cape May Lighthouse,
215 Light House Avenue, Cape May Point

B1 Village Bicycle Shop, 605 Lafayette Street, Cape May, NJ

BR1 Shields Bike Rentals,11 Gurney St, Cape May, NJ

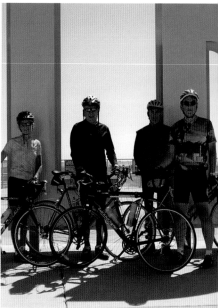
Thanks for the ride, David! Image courtesy David Wender.

23.0 Bear left to pick up Bayshore Dr.

23.4 Right on Sunset Blvd/Rt 606.

24.5 Left on Lighthouse Ave.

25.3 Arrive back at The Cape May Lighthouse.

The Cape May Lighthouse to Delaware Bay

Altitude ft

200

100

0

0   5   10   15   20   25.3

Distance miles

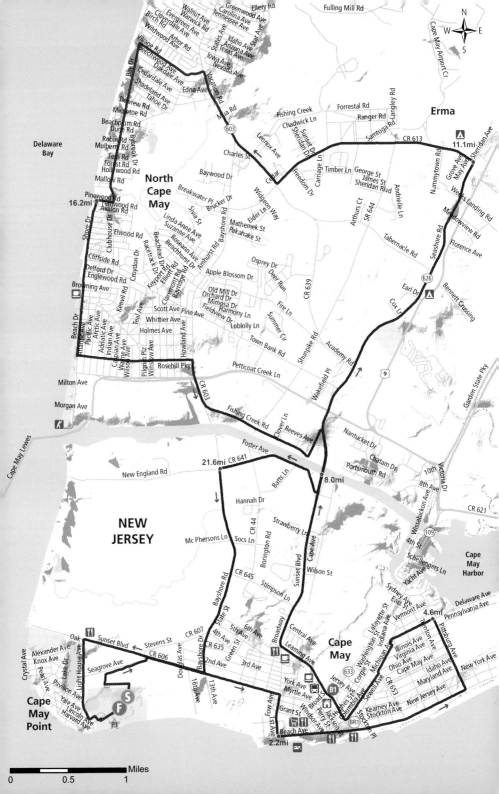

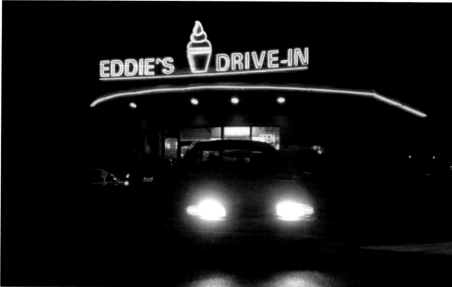

Eddie's in all its glory.

At a Glance

Distance 40.4 miles   **Total Elevation** 388 feet

Terrain

Delightful rolling hills on peaceful roads bring you along the river and through semi-rural areas, with a few little towns in between.

Traffic

There is little traffic on the long stretches of road during this ride, however, traffic picks up the closer you get to Phillipsburg and Easton. There is heavy traffic in Easton.

How to Get There

Frenchtown, New Jersey is about an hour and fifteen minutes drive from Philadelphia on Route 611. It's north of New Hope and Lambertville (Ride 33).

Food and Drink

The ride begins and ends at a little market, in case you want to grab a snack before or after the ride. There are also quite a few restaurants and cafés in Phillipsburg and Easton.

Side Trip

The Crayola Factory is in Easton! You'll ride right by the museum on 30 Centre Square. Make a stop and pop in to learn about how Crayola crayons and markers are made, and then draw all over the walls.

Where to Bike Rating

About...

The landscape of this route is very unique. As you travel from Frenchtown, New Jersey, to Easton, Pennsylvania, the ride winds through the woods and a few small towns, and then opens up into a huge swatch of land with soybeans and corn stalks. There are quite a lot of beautiful views of the Delaware River, which you'll crisscross time and again.

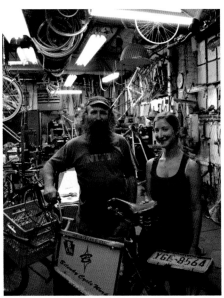

Bilenky in his shop with daughter, Bina.

These roads are just awesome for bicycles. There are really long stretches without turns, and, on most of the roads, there's little to get in your way in terms of traffic or potholes. You can burn them up or take a leisurely pedal and spend the day with your bicycle and a pal. If you want to check out this area but don't want to commit to a 40 mile loop, take the log to mile 8.4 and turn down Old River Road for a shorter 17 mile loop.

The ride begins in Frenchtown, New Jersey, and travels north to Easton, Pennsylvania on the New Jersey side of the Delaware River. Along the way, you'll bike through a bunch of small towns, including Milford and Holland. They all have a great look – old brick buildings and train stations call up a past bustling with manufacturing and industry.

After riding along the river between town and country, you'll come to Phillipsburg. The center of town has a great looking old cityscape; you may want to lock your bikes up and have a walk around or grab a snack at Eddie's Drive-in, just before the bridge.

When ready to leave, you'll cross the Phillipsburg-Easton Bridge to arrive in Easton. It's best to walk your bikes along the pedestrian walkways here. There are a lot of shops and restaurants in Easton, and definitely more traffic! So be careful as you make your way through town.

You'll ride on the Pennsylvania side of the river on your way back to Easton. There is a bit more traffic on the way home, so stick to single file riding on the right side of the road.

Thanks to Stephen Bilenky, a local frame builder in Philadelphia, who spent an afternoon showing me around these parts. We took our sweet time in early fall – it was still warm and the leaves were just beginning to change colors. An absolutely beautiful time of year for this ride!

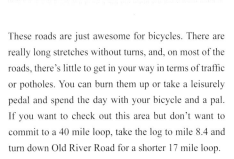

South Jersey

Ride Log.

 P1 Eddie's Drive-In, 4 Union Sq, Phillipsburg, NJ
P2 Crayola Factory,30 Centre Square, Easton, PA

 B1 Cycle Funattic,403 S Main St, Phillipsburg, NJ
B2 Genesis Bicycles, 126 Bushkill St, Easton, PA

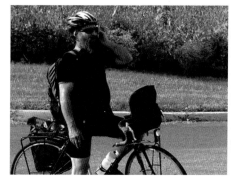

Bilenky takes a break.

0.0 Start at Frenchtown Market, on the corner of Sixth St and Milford Rd in Frenchtown, N.J. Bike west on Milford Rd.

0.4 Milford dead ends at 12th St. Make a left on 12th and then a quick right on Milford Frenchtown Rd.

3.3 Come to an intersection with Bridge and Water streets. Make a left on Bridge St.

3.4 Right on Church St.

3.5 Right on Spring Garden St (becomes River Rd, then Riegelsville Milford Rd).

8.4 Cross Old River Rd.

10.2 Road dead ends. Make a left on Riegelsville Warren Glen Rd.

10.3 Right to get back on River Rd. You'll be riding alongside the Conrail Railroad.

13.1 Cross Creek Rd to stay on River Rd.

15.3 River Rd ends. Make a right onto Carpentersville Rd.

17.8 Carpentersville Rd meets Rt 22. Make a left on Rt 22 and take it through Phillipsburg (there will be more traffic here).

20.0 Left on Rt. 248/S Main St to take the Northampton St Bridge over the Delaware River. Eddie's Drive-in is on the corner.

20.3 Come to the Center Square in Easton. Make a left on Third St.

20.6 Take the Third St/Smith Ave Bridge over the Le-

high River.

20.7 Left on Rt 611/S Delaware Dr. You'll ride on 611 for the next nine miles, almost all the way home!

29.3 Make a left on Delaware Rd.

29.4 Right on Durham St.

29.4 Left on Maplewood Rd. Take the bridge to cross the Delaware River yet again.

29.6 Right on River Rd, after the bridge (this will be familiar – mile marker 8.4).

29.7 Left on Riegelsville Warren Glen Rd.

29.8 Right on Riegelsville Milford Rd.

30.7 Right on Old River Rd and follow the bend to the left.

31.8 Right on Riegelsville Milford Rd (this becomes River Rd, then Spring Garden Rd).

36.9 Left on Church St.

37.0 Left on Bridge St.

37.1 Right on Frenchtown Rd, which becomes Milford Frenchtown Rd.

40.3 Left on Sixth St.

40.4 Arrive back at the Frenchtown Market.

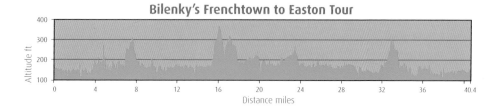

Bilenky's Frenchtown to Easton Tour

Distance miles

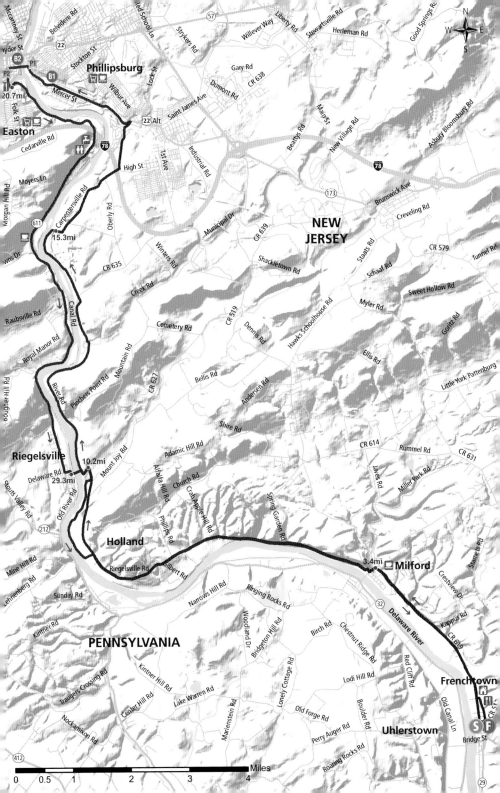

Kids' Rides

So, where do you go biking with a kiddo? This section introduces you to a few of the most enjoyable and safe places in the Philadelphia area to ride bikes with kids.

The first part of the section focuses solely on paths and parks in the city. You will be able to take public transit to all of these locations, and many are centrally located. Some of the parks are great for the littlest of riders, including Franklin Square (Ride K1), The Schuylkill River Park (Ride K2), The Azalea Garden (Ride K5), Clark Park (Ride K6), and Penn Treaty Park (Ride K13). A few offer longer trails, including MLK Drive (Ride K4), Pennypack Park (Ride K9), and FDR Park (Ride K11).

The second part of this section gives ideas for places to ride with kids in the suburbs. The majority of these rides are slightly longer than the ones in the city, and they offer a quiet suburban, rural, or beach vibe.

Of course, many of the adult rides are also suitable for tykes, just look for the Kid Friendly icon on the maps. Specifically, try out some of the State Parks and portions of the Schuylkill River Trail for a day of family fun. You won't be disappointed.

Happy Trails!

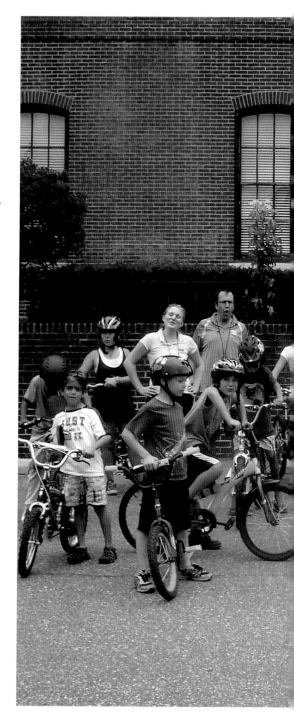

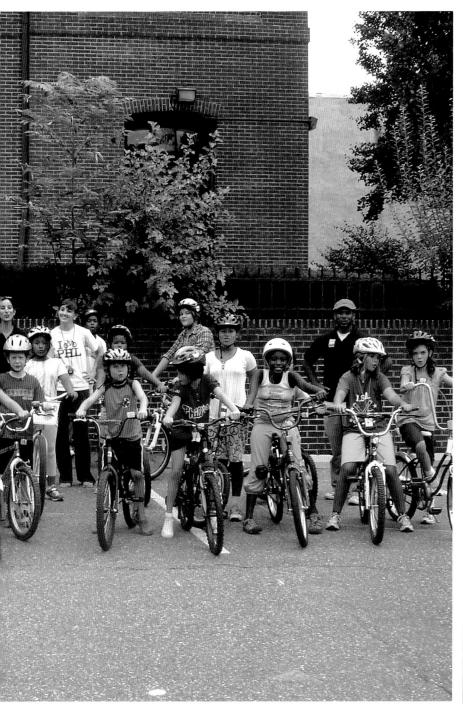

Safe Routes Philly. Photo courtesy Bicycle Coalition of Greater Philadelphia.

Kids' Rides

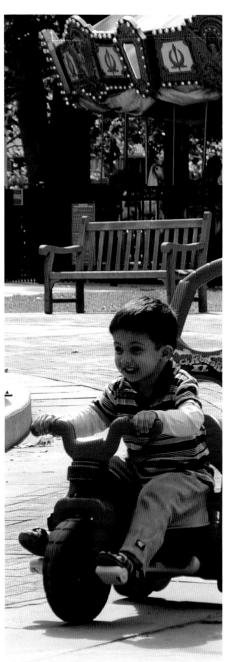

Distance 0.3 miles

Terrain

Franklin Square has a flat circular path that goes around the carousel. There's also a small enclosed playground next to the fountain.

How to Get There

Located on Sixth and Race, the square is within easy walking distance of Center City. The 47 bus will drop you nearby, and there is parking around The Constitution Center.

Amenities and Things to Do

There is so much to do in Franklin Square! When the little ones tire of their wheels, you can throw coins into the marble fountain, have an ice cream at Square Burger, run around the playground, listen to the Once Upon a Nation storyteller, or ride the classic carousel.

About

In the late 17th century, William Penn set aside Franklin Square as one of the five open-space parks he planned for the city. Today it is a very friendly and comfortable park, and it makes for an especially good spot for the little tykes on bikes.

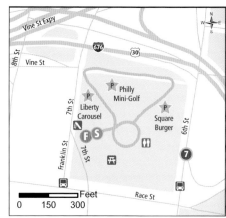

Riding around the fountain at Franklin Square.

Ride K2 - The Schuylkill River Park

Distance 0.2 miles

Terrain

There is a series of paved walkways and an enclosed recreation area for the kiddos.

How to Get There

The entrance to the park is on 25th Street between Pine and Spruce in Center City, with street parking along 25th. Buses 7, 12, and 40 serve the area.

Amenities and Things to Do

Between its basketball and tennis courts, enclosed dog run, community garden, and totally happenin' playground, there is always a lot of activity in this park. On Wednesday afternoons in season, you'll find a small farmers' market too!

About

The Schuylkill River Park is a great neighborhood spot. Its walkways are good for kids, and the little ones can feel free buzzing about on bikes, trikes, and scooters in the enclosed recreation area. One hitch on the rec area – the big kids take over on Wednesday evenings and Sunday afternoons for rousing matches of Bike Polo.

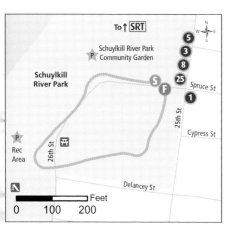

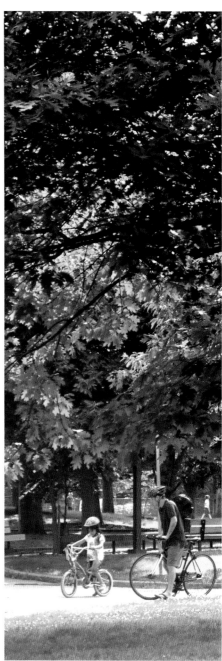

Look dad! No more training wheels!

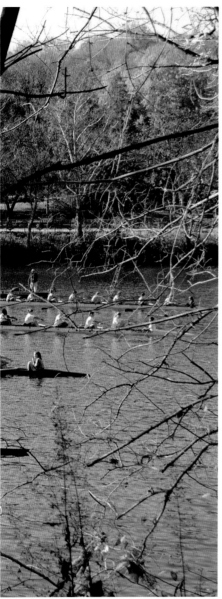

Crews getting ready to race.

P1 Regatta Grandstand
P2 Playing Angels Statue

Distance 0.8 miles, 1.6 miles round trip

Terrain

This section of the loop is an enjoyable, flat path that runs along the Schuylkill River.

How to Get There

There is parking next to the Girard Bridge and the Columbia Bridge. You can also walk from the Boathouse Row area.

Amenities and Things to Do

Picnic tables along the banks and patches of lush green grass are perfect for sunny afternoons and counting crews row up and down the river. The grandstand for watching Sunday regattas is just below the Columbia Bridge.

About

The Schuylkill River Trail is always packed with bicycle and pedestrian traffic. Families and kids are welcome everywhere, but the stretch between the Girard Bridge and the Columbia Bridge has an extra gravel path that runs alongside the main trail. It alleviates some of the congestion and can be a great option for kids.

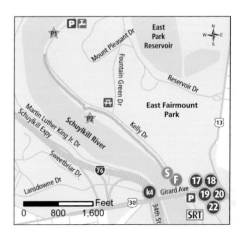

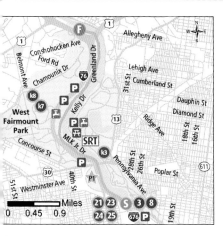

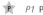 **P1** Philadelphia Zoo

istance 3.9 miles, 6.8 miles round trip

errain

1LK Drive is a wide, flat thruway on the west side of
1e Schuylkill River.

low to Get There

ollow directions as you would to the Art Museum or
toathouse Row. You can pick up MLK Drive at the
ntersection of Schuylkill Banks Park and Ben Franklin
arkway. Take the Ben Franklin Parkway bridge to
1e west side of the river. You'll have to ride on the
idewalk for a short while before the drive begins.

menities and Things to Do

he main draw here is the fact that this huge road is
losed to traffic on the weekends in the summer. Enjoy it!

bout

ormerly West River Drive, MLK is closed to most
ars on weekends in the summer. It's great for kids
ig and small, and it's such a popular destination that
ou're bound to catch a familiar face or two. There's
lso a path that runs between the drive and the river, in
ase you'd like to hop out here during the week.

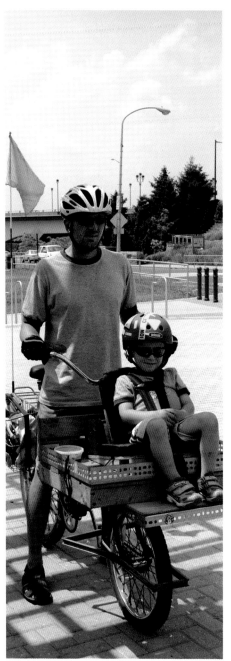

Travis & Owen getting ready to roll.

City Kids' Rides

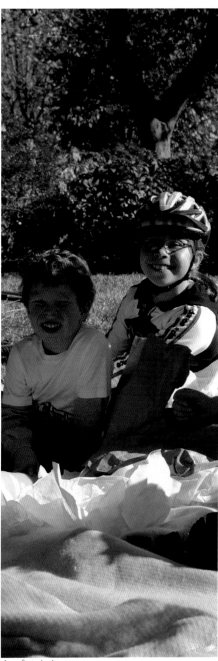

A perfect picnic.

Distance 0.4 miles

Terrain

The easy path through the four acre Azalea Garden is flat and paved.

How to Get There

The garden is on the grounds of the Philadelphia Museum of Art. It is easily accessed by the parking lot behind Lloyd Hall.

Amenities and Things to Do

This is a picturesque spot for a picnic, especially in the spring. (According to the Fairmount Park Commission, the garden contains over 150 species of azaleas and rhododendrons). It is also very close to other places you might want to explore, including Boathouse Row and the Water Works.

About

The area around the Azalea Garden is often less crowded than some of the other spots by Kelly Drive and is partially secluded from the street, giving little tykes more freedom to pedal. Enjoy this island oasis of lush grass and scattered shade!

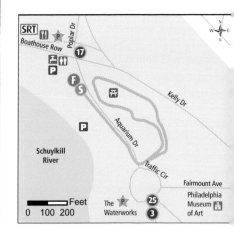

istance 0.6 miles

errain

lark Park is a city playground and park with short aved paths running throughout.

ow to Get There

he park is located between 43rd and 45th streets, and altimore Avenue and Woodland Avenue, in West niladelphia. There are two sections, with Chester venue running between. The trolley will bring you irectly to the park, and the 30 bus will drop you off lose by.

menities and Things to Do

lark Park is great for picnicking and relaxing, with a layground for the little guys too. If you're lucky, the upcake Lady will drive her multi-colored truck by for n afternoon sugar high.

bout

stablished in 1895, Clark Park offers over nine acres f green space to the University City community. It's n the smaller side, so probably best for the tiny bikes nd trikes. Annual festivals, flea markets, and a seasonal rmers' market all add to the positive vibe here. Check ut www.friendsofclarkpark.org for more info.

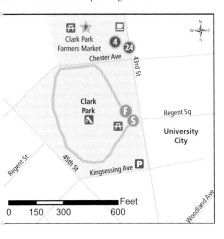

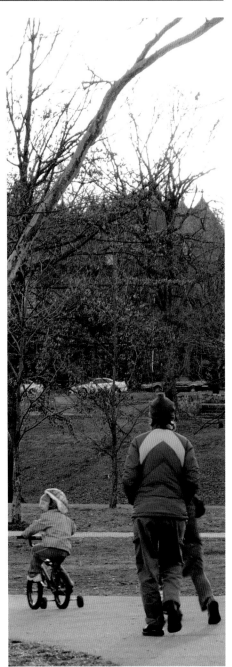

Late afternoon on a cool winter's day in Clark Park.

City Kids' Rides

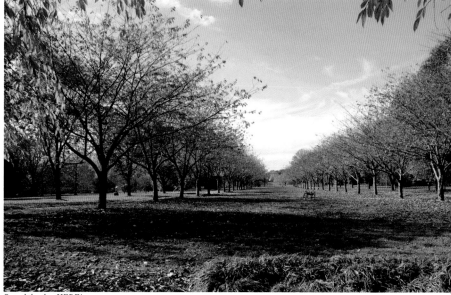

Spend the day HERE!

Distance 0.6 miles, 1.2 miles round trip

Terrain

Among a network of paths, you'll find a bike lane near the entrance to the Horticulture Center and a small loop around the gazebo.

How to Get There

The center is located at North Horticultural Drive and Montgomery Avenue in Fairmount Park. Septa buses 38, 40, 43 and 64 stop nearby, and in the summer the Phlash Downtown Loop stops by The Please Touch Museum. There is also a small parking area behind the center.

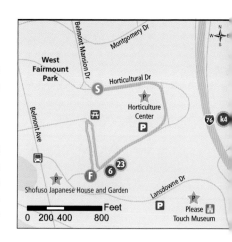

Amenities and Things to Do

The Horticulture Center has beautiful sculptures, a reflecting pool and a number of display gardens including the 20 acre Centennial Arboretum. The Japanese Tea House is across the street, and the Please Touch Museum is just around the corner.

About

Wind your way through the exotic trees and butterfl gardens in this section of Fairmount Park – there ar quiet paths for the little guys and miles more to explor for bigger kids. It's not far from Center City an definitely worth the trip!

istance 1.0 miles, 2.0 miles round trip

errain

his comfortable paved path runs adjacent to
hamounix Drive, conveniently separated from the
reet by a median.

ow to Get There

hamounix Drive is located in West Fairmount Park.
he 38 and 40 buses will drop you within walking
istance of Chamounix Mansion, which is at the end
f the drive. There are a few large parking lots nearby
s well.

menities and Things to Do

he drive is peppered with sports fields, tennis
ourts, and picnic areas. Both the historic Chamounix
Mansion, built in 1802, and the Chamounix Equestrian
Center are located at the end of the drive.

bout

hamounix Drive is a great option for a relaxed
ummer afternoon! Most of the path is shaded, and
here are tons of recreational opportunities nearby if
our kiddo is maxed out on pedaling. Of course if you
ant to increase mileage, Chamounix is hooked into a
reater network of lanes around Fairmount.

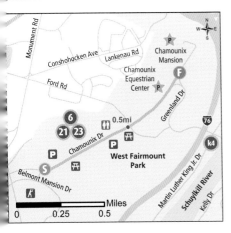

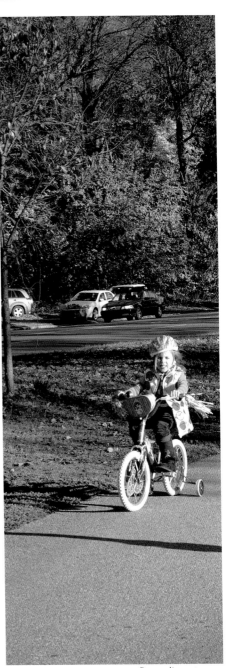

Best cycling getup ever.

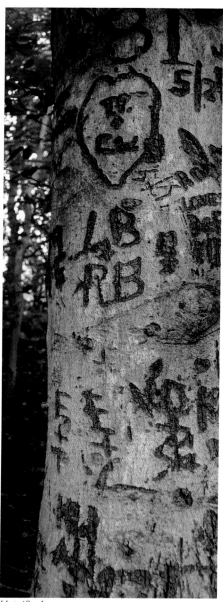

LL + AS = Love.

⭐ **P** *P1* Fox Chase Farm
P2 Pennypack Environmental Center

Distance 4.0 miles, 8.0 miles round trip

Terrain

A few short, steep hills make this curvy gravel pat
along the Pennypack Creek a fun adventure for kid
on wheels! There are also a lot of hidden MBT path
through the woods.

How to Get There

Pennypack is located in Northeast Philadelphia. The 6
bus will drop you at Verree Road and Tustin Stree
and the 58 at Bustleton and Winchester Avenue – bot
a stone's throw from trail entrances. There is ampl
parking at the trail head off Shady Lane.

Amenities and Things to Do

Oh lots! There are summer concerts here on Wednesda
evenings, fun spots for fishing if you don't mind no
catching a fish, and cool old bridges to explore. Plus
Pennypack is chock full of birds, geese, turtles, an
deer.

About

While Pennypack stretches on for seven miles, the
four between Shady Lane and Bustleton are my
favorites for kids. The hills will have them yelling
wheeeeeeeeeeeeee all the way home!

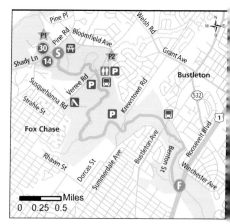

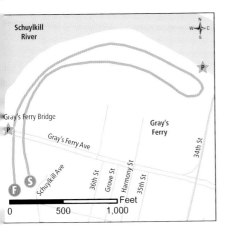

Distance 1.0 miles

Terrain

The Gray's Ferry Crescent is a new path along the Schuylkill River, set to be completed in spring 2011.

How to Get There

The entrance to the path is just under the Gray's Ferry Avenue Bridge on the east side of the Schuylkill River. Buses 12 and 64 will drop you near the entrance.

About

The completion of the Gray's Ferry Crescent will create a new strip of greenspace in this part of the city. Eventually, it will connect to the Locust Street entrance of the Schuylkill River Trail (Ride 3), extending recreational opportunities along the river.

A recent success of the Complete the River Trail Campaign, the Gary's Ferry Crescent is a nifty little path between the 34th Street/University Avenue Bridge and Gray's Ferry Avenue Bridge. Stay tuned for more trail connections!

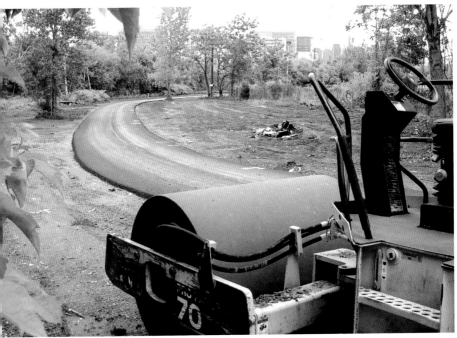

Gray's Ferry Crescent on its way!

City Kids' Rides

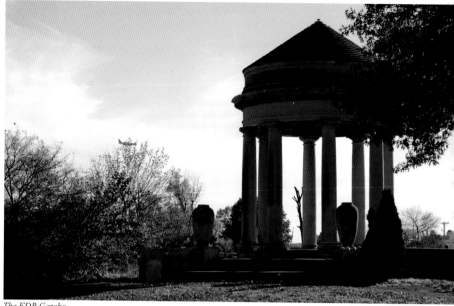

The FDR Gazebo.

Distance 1.7 miles

Terrain

The loop around FDR Park is a paved, multipurpose path with steady bicycle and pedestrian traffic.

How to Get There

FDR is near the stadiums in South Philadelphia. The 17 and 71 buses will drop you off at Broad and Pattison, or you can take the Broad Street subway to Pattison Avenue – you'll find an entrance to the park on the corner. There is parking here as well.

Amenities and Things to Do

In addition to the bike path, you'll find a golf course, fields for baseball and rugby, tennis courts, and the well known FDR Skate Park. What a gem!

About

The path goes around the lagoon in the middle of the

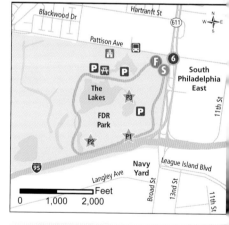

 P1 FDR Skate Park
P2 Baseball Fields
P3 Meadow Lake

park, which, with a few other waterways here, gives FDR its nickname, "The Lakes". There are some smaller paths that cut across the main loop that you might want to explore as well.

Ride K12 - Delaware River Trail (Pier 70)

Distance 0.7 miles, 1.4 miles round trip

Terrain

This new path (dedicated May 27th, 2010!) features the Delaware River to the east and shopping to the west. Because it is so new and so lightly traveled, the path is very well paved.

How to Get There

Buses 7, 25, 29, and 64 will all drop you in the Wal-Mart parking lot. The trail seriously starts right behind the store.

Amenities and Things to Do

You'll enjoy nice views of that other huge river in the city – The Delaware. There are a couple of pleasant spots for watching the ships and boats, and some great city views too.

About

The Pier 70 Trail is short and sweet – it is the first section of the Delaware River Trail, which could one day stretch from Pier 70 to Allegheny Avenue. Oh what a beautiful vision!

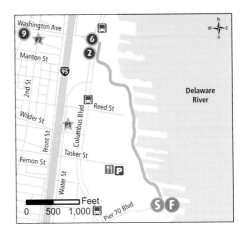

 P1 Riverview Plaza Stadium 17 (Movies)
P2 Mummer's Museum

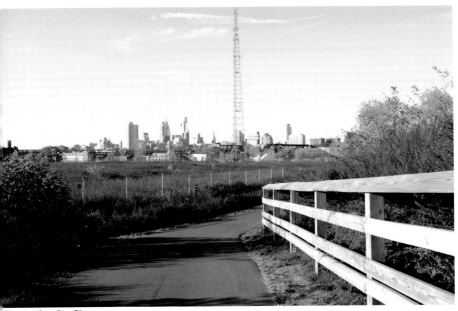

The view from Pier 70.

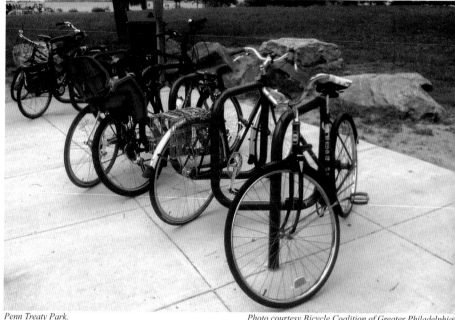

Penn Treaty Park.   *Photo courtesy Bicycle Coalition of Greater Philadelphia*

Distance 0.3 miles

Terrain

Penn Treaty Park is a small park on the banks of the Delaware River. There is a short path that wraps around the trees and picnic benches.

How to Get There

The park is located in the Fishtown section of Philadelphia, just off North Delaware Avenue and East Columbia Avenue. The 43 bus will drop you directly at the park, and the 25 will bring you a few blocks south.

Amenities and Things to Do

Watch the boats along the Delaware, hop on the playground, and enjoy a summer picnic! A number of annual festivals also take place here, including Shadfest in the spring, and flea markets, dog days and concerts in the summer.

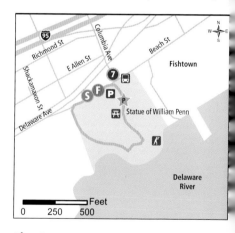

About

Penn Treaty Park commemorates the friendship treaty signed between William Penn and the Leni Lenape Native Americans in the late 17th Century. The park officially opened in 1893 and remains today a happy meeting place for many Philadelphians.

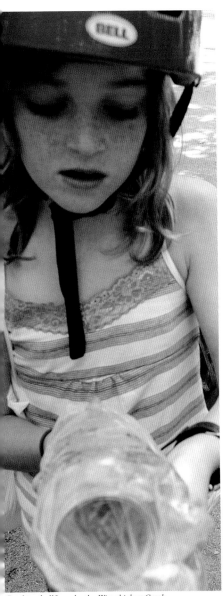

Catching bullfrogs by the Wissahickon Creek.

P1 Wissahickon Creek
P2 Morris Arboretum

Distance 1.7 miles, 3.4 miles round trip

Terrain

The Wissahickon Valley Park is gravel in some places and paved in others.

How to Get There

The park is close to Exit 26 on the PA Turnpike. There is parking by Militia Hill and the Flourtown day use area.

Amenities and Things to Do

You'll find playgrounds, ballparks, and picnic areas along the trail. The ride also winds along the Wissahickon Creek, which is great for fishing, catching frogs and spying other wildlife. There are over 60 species of butterflies here, including swallowtails, hairstreaks, harvesters, and skippers!

About

Just up the road is the famous Fort Washington State Park named for the temporary fort that George Washington established here during the American Revolution. Over 12,000 soldiers stayed here for six weeks in the early winter of 1777, before marching to Valley Forge.

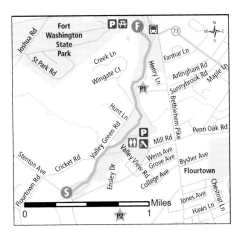

Suburbs Kids' Rides

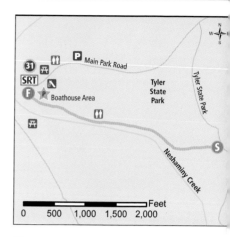

Distance 0.6 miles, 1.2 miles round trip

Terrain

Tyler Drive is a flat, multi-use paved path through the state park.

How to Get There

Septa bus 130 will drop you at Bucks County Community College. Otherwise, pack up your zipcar and head for the hills!

Amenities and Things to Do

There are over 1700 acres of farm and woodlands in Tyler State Park. The section of the Neshaminy Creek by the main pavilion is the perfect place to fish or get your feet wet. You'll find plenty of picnic areas scattered throughout the park as well.

About

There are over 10 bicycle trails in Tyler State Park, but the straight and relatively flat Tyler Drive Trail near the boathouse area is a good choice for kids. It is shaded and cool, and its straight path along the creek means that you can turn around at anytime.

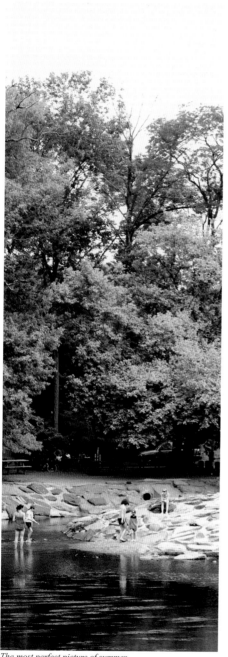

The most perfect picture of summer.

Distance
4.3 miles, 8.6 miles round trip

Terrain
Peace Valley has a couple of multi-use paths that run about half of the way around Lake Galena. The paved bike/hike path includes Creek Road and New Galena Road.

How to Get There
Peace Valley is north of Philadelphia in New Britain, Bucks County. Not a ton of good public transit options up this way, so you'll most likely have to pack up the car for the afternoon. The entrance is just off Callowhill Road and New Galena Road.

Amenities and Things to Do
Be sure to check out the Peace Valley Nature Center, which offers unique environmental education programs year 'round.

About
Play all day long! With over 1500 acres, Peace Valley offers opportunities for hiking, picnicking, fishing, and boating. And the warm summer months bring fun special events – the fishing derbies and environmental treasure hunts top the list!

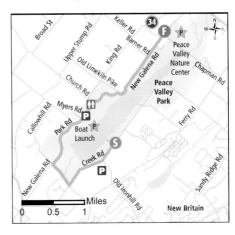

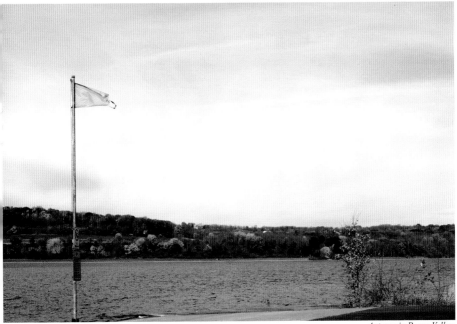

Autumn in Peace Valley.

Suburbs
Kids' Rides

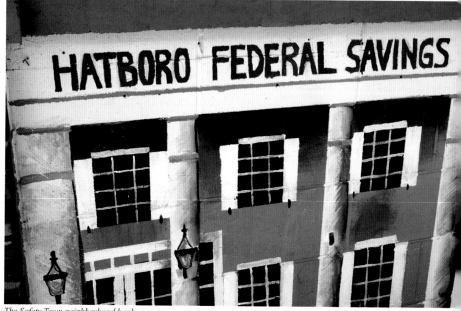

The Safety Town neighborhood bank.

Distance 0.2 miles

Terrain

Oh geez, this place is adorable. The "terrain" is an enclosed "street" for kids on tricycles and d-scooters, complete with traffic lights.

How to Get There

Mason's Mill is located north of the city, in Huntington Valley. The 55 bus will take a while, but it will drop you within walking distance of the park.

Amenities and Things to Do

Mason's Mill Park has a little bit of everything – basketball and tennis courts, softball fields, shady walking paths, playgrounds, and one awesome water fountain shaped like a cartoon lion's head.

About

Safety Town, where I spent many an afternoon as a kiddo, felt like a big city when I was three. Your tykes will roll by Senator Greenleaf's Headquarters, Hatboro Federal Savings, and The Willow Grove Fire Company, and other handpainted kiddo sized buildings. For the bigger ones, a ¾ mile trail loops the park.

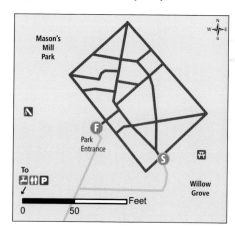

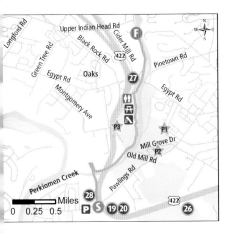

P1 John James Audubon Center
    1201 Pawlings Rd, Mill Grove
P2 Audubon Wildlife Sanctuary
P3 Lower Perkiomen Valley Park

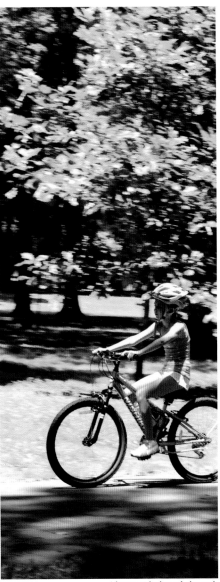

Distance 2.4 miles, 4.8 miles round trip

Terrain

The trail is paved until Upper Indian Road, and then it becomes packed gravel. There are some steep hills on Audubon Loop, which is nearby enough to wander onto by mistake.

How to Get There

You can bike out here via the Schuylkill River Trail! The park is just past Valley Forge. Of course, you can also drive – the entrance is close to Route 422 and New Mill Road and there is plenty of parking.

Amenities and Things to Do

This park is a ways from the city but offers a host of activities, including summer concerts, fishing, volleyball, barbeque grills, and a big grassy playground.

About

The path, which follows the Perkiomen Creek, is very family friendly; this park sees a ton of bicycle traffic. Plus, you can rent a pavilion for a birthday party and other summer celebrations!

A breezy ride through the park.

Suburbs
Ki s' Ri es

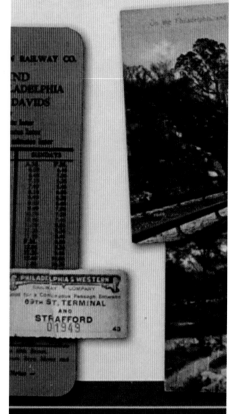

ore profitable. In it
ity opposition and
l overgrown. After
l opened in 2005.

left: P&W schedules from
right: Postcards like these
o Main Line residents who

Sign welcoming you to Radnor Trail.

Distance 2.4 miles, 4.8 miles round trip

Terrain

The Radnor Trail is a paved, multi-use path along the old Philadelphia and Western Railway.

How to Get There

The trail is located in Wayne, west of Philadelphia on the Mainline. It runs between Radnor-Chester Road and Sugartown Road, with parking on Brookside Avenue. It's also possible to walk from Strafford station, a stop on the Paoli/Thorndale Regional Rail line.

Amenities and Things to Do

There are lots of trees and quiet places for a rest or picnic on the Radnor Trail, but beware, there is not a single restroom for 2.4 miles!

About

The old P & W Railway connected the 69th Street Terminal and Strafford until 1956. In 2005, the Radnor Trail opened as a classic "Rails to Trails" project. A great option for families, the path winds between wooded and residential areas, and it is shady and green.

P1 Encke Park

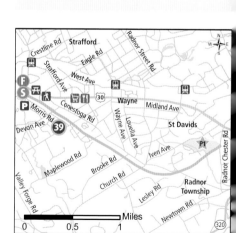

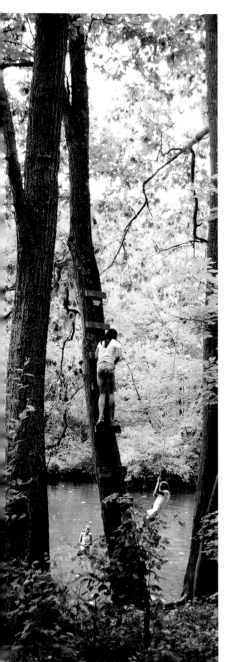

Swinging into the Brandywine.

P1 Kardon Park
P2 Uwchlan Trail

Distance 2.5 miles, 5.0 miles round trip

Terrain

The Struble Trail is a shaded, paved path that curves along the Brandywine Creek.

How to Get There

Hoof it on out to Chester County! It's a drive. Parking is located just off the trail head on Norwood Road.

Amenities and Things to Do

The creek is the big attraction here – there are wonderful and giant trees to swing from, sandy banks to jump off of, and oodles of critters to catch. Don't forget your swimsuit for a dip in the creek during the warmer months!

About

Families and kids of all ages bike, stroll, run, and play along the Struble year 'round. The path is very well maintained, and it's surrounded by a thin forest. A little bonus – Victory Brewing is nearby, just in case Mom or Dad need a rest.

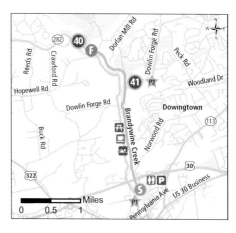

Distance 2.7 miles

Terrain
The wide bike lanes in Beach Haven are on slow side streets. You will see lots of families and children of all ages enjoying these paths.

How to Get There
Pack the bikes and drive east. There is parking all over the island.

Amenities and Things to Do
When you get tired of pedaling, you can take a dip in the ocean (lifeguards are stationed on beaches all along the island), have an ice cream, or visit the ferris wheel in the middle of town. It's a great place to spend a summer afternoon or weekend.

 P1 Surflight Theater

About
A Jersey Shore biking mecca! There is an excellen network of bike lanes in Beach Haven, which is located on the southern end of Long Beach Island. You can also rent bikes for kids and adults at shops all over th island. Check out Ride 48 for more information about biking on LBI.

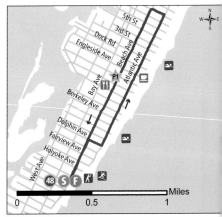

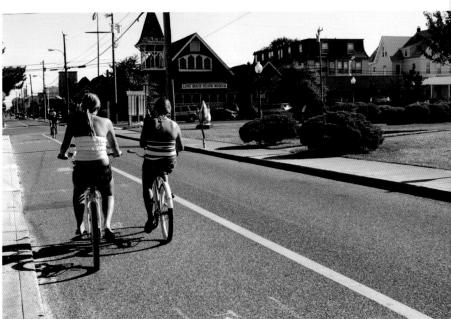

Summer freedom!

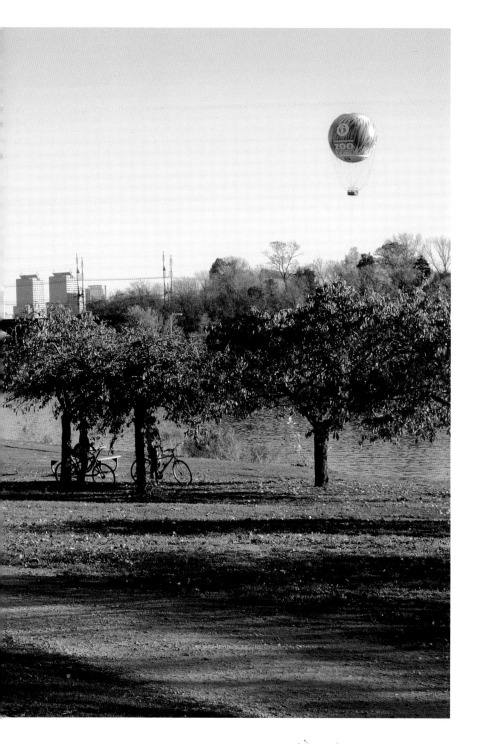

Notes

Notes

Notes

Notes

Notes

Notes

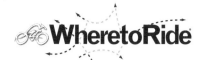 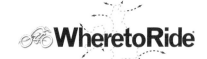

Also in this **Series!**

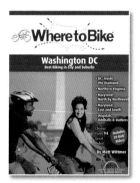 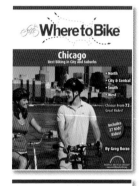 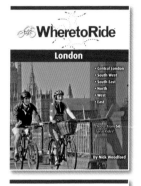

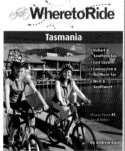 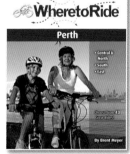 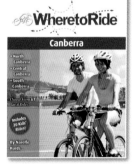

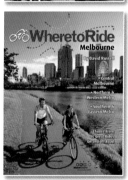 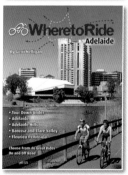

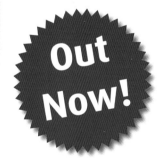

www.**WheretoBikeGuides**.com

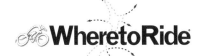 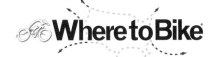
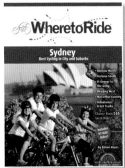
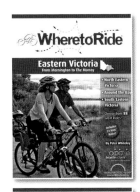
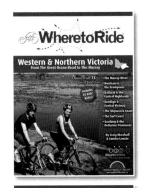
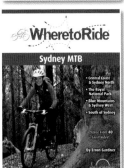
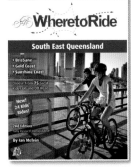
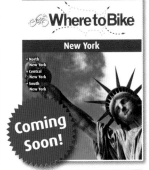
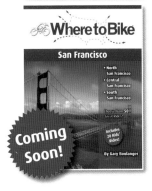
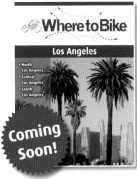
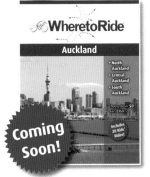

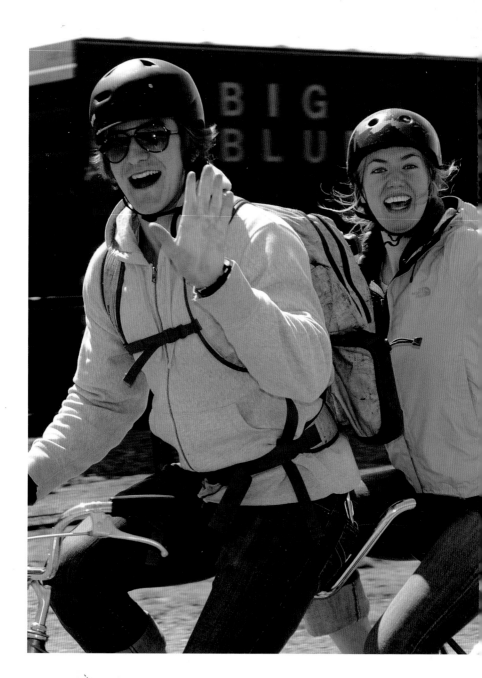